Colour **Aids**

Rheumatology

J. M. H. Moll BSc DM PhD FRCP

Consultant Physician in
Rheumatology, Nether Edge Hospital,
Sheffield; Head, Sheffield Centre for
Rheumatic Diseases; Honorary
Clinical Lecturer in Rheumatic
Diseases, University of Sheffield

Churchill Livingstone

EDINBURGH LONDON MELBOURNE AND NEW YORK 1984

Preface

In general, rheumatology is a specialty eminently suited to pictorial representation. Surface colour changes and alterations in the morphology of the limbs and trunk combine to form a myriad of unique clinical patterns. Once seen, these are rarely forgotten.

The source of this collection is largely personal and was started some 20 years ago when the author was a house physician. Here and there, however, it has been necessary to take advantage of the kind cooperation of the following colleagues to provide slides of rarities or simply to fill gaps created by lost or unrecognised clinical opportunity: Dr R. S. Amos, Dr N. A. Barrington, Dr M. J. Brown, Dr G. N. Chandler, Dr D. Cumberland, Dr M. S. Derini, Mr R. A. Elson, the late Dr H. G. Garland, Dr F. D. Hart, Dr P. Hughes, Dr G. R. Newns, Dr N. R. Rowell, Professor R. G. G. Russell, the late Dr R. N. Tattersall, Dr J. Winfield, Professor V. Wright.

I also wish to thank my secretary, Mrs Pat Drake for typing the manuscript and the publishers for guidance in its presentation.

Sheffield   J. M. H. M.

Contents

1 | Rheumatoid Arthritis (RA) (1)

Definition

Chronic polyarthritis characterised by bilateral symmetrical joint disease, radiological erosions, positive tests for rheumatoid factor and, pathologically, a chronic proliferative synovitis with villous hypertrophy, infiltration by lymphocytes and plasma cells, and by nodules. It is a multisystem disorder, justifying the use by some of the term 'rheumatoid *disease*'. The condition is often included under the systemic connective tissue diseases (collagenoses). Diagnostic criteria are available.

Prevalence

Affects 6% females and 2% of males. World-wide distribution. The most common inflammatory disease of joints in UK (affecting about 1.5×10^6) and elsewhere. Onset: 16–70 yr; most often: 20–55 yr.

Aetiology

The cause is unknown. A prominent feature is the formation of immune complexes within the joint. These activate complement and attract neutrophils. Phagocytosis of immune complexes by neutrophils leads to release of chemical mediators of inflammation. Continued inflammation stimulates the formation of a proliferative synovitis. This hypertrophic granulation tissue is called pannus (Fig. 1). It is this that is responsible for causing joint erosions. These can be seen clearly as macroscopic lesions on the joint surface (Fig. 1) or on X-ray (Fig. 2).

Fig. 1 RA. Synovial hypertrophy and erosions of articular cartilage.

Fig. 2 RA. Periarticular erosions of MCP joints.

Clinical features: joint disease

Hands

A typical onset is the appearance of pain, stiffness (usually early morning stiffness), swelling and tenderness of the knuckle joints—proximal interphalangeal (PIPs) and metacarpophalangeal (MCPs). Fusiform swelling of the PIP joints gives the fingers a characteristic spindle shape (Fig. 3). With more advanced disease MCP subluxation and ulnar deviation of the fingers occurs (Fig. 4), and also boutonnière and swan-neck deformities (Fig. 5). The wrists are also often involved. This feature, together with the absence of distal interphalangeal (DIP) involvement with Heberden's nodes, helps to differentiate rheumatoid arthritis (RA) of the hands from that other common arthropathy—osteoarthrosis (OA). If Bouchard's nodes (OA of PIP joints) are present they are differentiated as hard swellings, compared with the softer joint swelling in rheumatoid arthritis. However, as both are common diseases they may co-exist. Psoriatic arthritis will usually be obvious because of the asymmetry and oligoarticular pattern of involvement, apart from the presence of skin and/ or nail involvement. Gout barely comes into the differential diagnosis as it causes severe inflammatory features, and in some patients tophi will make the diagnosis clear. Carcinoma arthritis may be indistinguishable from rheumatoid arthritis.

Fig. 3 Early RA. Synovial thickening of PIP joints and wrists. Deformity minimal.

Fig. 4 RA at later stage. Considerable MCP joint thickening, subluxation and ulnar deviation.

Fig. 5 Advanced RA. Swan-neck deformities and synovial thickening of wrists.

**Clinical
features:
joint
disease**
(contd)

Feet
Irritable MTP joints are the main source of
trouble. Patients feel as though there are pebbles
in their shoe. On examination calluses may be
seen over these joints (Fig. 6), and the counterpart
deformities to those seen in the hand may be
obvious (Figs 6 & 7)—fibular deviation of the toes.
Other features may be present including
discharging fistulae (Fig. 8).

Other joints
Progression of the disease may result in spread to
almost all peripheral joints. The spine (limited to
the upper cervical region) may be involved.
Although less common, even the arytenoid joints
(synovial joints) may become affected.

**Clinical
features:
soft-tissue
rheumatic
manifesta-
tions**

1. Bursal swellings and rupture
An important complication is the enlargement
and rupture of bursal cysts near joints. Notable is
popliteal (Baker's) cyst rupture causing leakage of
synovial fluid from the knee into the calf. This
may be diagnosed erroneously as a deep vein
thrombosis. In the patient shown in Fig. 9 the cyst
had become infected.

Fig. 6 RA. Calluses over subluxated MTP joints and fibular deviation of toes.

Fig. 7 RA. Marked hallux valgus and fibular deviation of other toes.

Fig. 8 RA. Healing fistula had been discharging synovial fluid from ankle joint.

Fig. 9 RA. Ruptured Baker's cyst with massive calf extension containing pus.

Clinical features: soft-tissue rheumatic manifestations (contd)

2. Diseases of tendons and tendon sheaths
Rupture of an extensor tendon or tendons may occur due to the destructive effect of synovial proliferation and roughened bones on the dorsum of the wrist. Extensor tendon rupture manifests as a 'dropped finger' with inability to extend the digit, and there is usually prominent synovial thickening on the dorsum of the wrist (Fig. 10). This diagnosis is important, as splintage to encourage natural union or surgical repair is often beneficial.

Rupture of a flexor tendon or tendons may occur due to the same effect on the palmar aspect of the wrist. This presents as an inability to bend the finger. Prominent synovial bulging is usually also evident on the front of the wrist (Fig. 11).

Trigger finger may occur due to tendon sheath involvement when the patient is unable to straighten the finger spontaneously (Fig. 12). A tendon or tendon sheath nodule may be palpable in the affected area.

Tendon or tendon sheath complications and associated deformities should not be confused with finger deformities due to interphalangeal (IP) joint disease (Fig. 13).

Fig. 10 RA. Extensor tendon rupture. Note swelling on back of wrist.

Fig. 11 RA. Flexor tendon rupture. Note swelling on front of wrist.

Fig. 12 RA. 'Trigger finger' due to tendon sheath nodule.

Fig. 13 RA. Clawed fingers due to rapidly progressive arthritis of PIP joints.

Clinical features: soft-tissue rheumatic manifestations (contd)

3. Nerve entrapment syndromes
Most common is the carpal tunnel syndrome which may occur at any stage in rheumatoid arthritis (see p. 91).

Clinical features: systemic manifestations

1. General
Weight loss, low-grade fever, lymph node enlargement, oedema, anaemia, osteoporosis (and fractures), infections and amyloidosis.

2. Arteritis
This is an indication of severe disease. In the fingers it gives rise to nail-fold infarcts—small brown/black marks (Fig. 14) which are often unnoticed by the patient. These may also occur elsewhere on the fingers (Fig. 15). More extensive arteritis is manifest by more obvious lesions, and even by extensive areas of gangrene (Fig. 16)—in this instance, after the gangrenous finger tips were sloughed, they 'regenerated' (including reformation of the nail) although the fingers were shorter than before. Infarcts may also occur in relation to rheumatoid nodules (see p. 11), and a typical example is shown in Fig. 17.

Fig. 14 RA. Nail fold, nail bed and dermal infarcts. (White nails incidental.)

Fig. 15 RA. Dermal infarcts (resembling small pigmented naevi).

Fig. 16 RA. Advanced digital gangrene with demarcation lines.

Fig. 17 RA. Dermal infarcts overlying elbow nodules.

Clinical features systemic manifesta-tions (contd)

3. Subcutaneous nodules
These are painless fleshy lumps varying from the size of a pea to that of a tangerine (0.5–3 cm diameter). Found typically over the olecranon (Figs 18 & 19), but may also be found over other bony prominences (e.g. bridge of nose, occiput, sacrum), or arising from tendons (particularly the tendo Achilles). They may also occur more 'deeply', and their appearance in the lungs (in patients with pneumoconiosis) is termed Caplan's syndrome (Fig. 20). Rheumatoid nodules only occur in patients with positive tests for rheumatoid factor (often highly positive) and are virtually diagnostic of the disorder.

4. Myelopathy and neuropathy
Although caused by different mechanisms, these neurological complications may be included here. Severe arthritis of the mid and upper cervical spine may cause damage to the cervical cord, presenting as tetraparesis or even tetraplegia. The spinal arthritis is usually considerable and associated with subluxation (Fig. 21). Neuropathy, either mononeuritis multiplex or polyneuropathy, is another neurological manifestation of severe systemic rheumatoid arthritis.

Fig. 18 RA. Small/medium sized elbow nodules.

Fig. 19 RA. Large nodules over distal ulna and in olecranon bursa.

Fig. 20 Caplan's syndrome. Massive rheumatoid nodules in both pneumoconiotic lung fields.

Fig. 21 RA. Severe mid-cervical spondylopathy with inter-vertebral subluxation anteriorly.

Clinical features: systemic manifestations (contd)

5. Eye disease
Several ocular manifestations are seen in this type of arthritis. The most common is episcleritis (Fig. 22). This is usually asymptomatic. More serious is scleritis (Fig. 22). The gravest ocular complication is scleromalacia perforans. This results in immediate and permanent blindness.

6. Other 'systemic' manifestations
Ulceration of the skin, usually over the sacrum (Fig. 23) or on the legs, is due to large-vessel arteritis. Another surface feature is palmar erythema (Fig. 24), and it is important not to assume liver disease from this sign in rheumatoid patients. Other systemic features are mentioned under the related syndromes (Sjögren's syndrome, p. 15; Felty's syndrome, p. 17).

Radiological features

Early: juxta-articular osteoporosis, erosions (see Fig. 2).
Late: loss of joint space, bone destruction and subluxation (see Fig. 21).

Laboratory features

Anaemia and raised ESR in active disease. Positive tests for rheumatoid factor (e.g. latex, Rose–Waaler). ANF often positive, LE cells present in 10%. Anti-DNA antibodies not present. HLA Dw4 and HLA DRw4 present in over 50%. Synovial fluid: turbid, yellow/green, low viscosity, clot-positive, approx. 30 000 WBC ($\times 10^9$/dl)—all characteristics of a 'non-specific' inflammatory exudate. (Gout and pseudogout fluids contain crystals, and the fluid of septic arthritis is culture-positive.)

Management

Advice/instruction; drugs: non-steroidal anti-inflammatory drugs at first—supplement, if necessary, with small-dose corticosteroids and/or a remission-inducing agent (e.g. gold, penicillamine or antimalarials); rest; exercises; aids and appliances; surgery.

Fig. 22 RA. Episcleritis right eye. Episcleritis + scleritis left eye.

Fig. 23 RA. Deep ulcer surrounded by healing ulcers.

Fig. 24 RA. Palmar erythema.

2 | Sjögren's Syndrome

Definition

Sjögren's syndrome (after Henrick S.C. Sjögren, b.1899) is a triad of defective lacrimal secretion (kerato-conjunctivitis sicca), defective salivary secretion (xerostomia), and a systemic connective tissue disorder. The term sicca syndrome is applied when the only features are dry eyes and mouth.

Prevalence

Most often seen in rheumatoid arthritis, 30% of whom show features of the syndrome. F : M; 9 : 1.

Aetiology

Immunological and immunogenetic factors have been reported. May be more than one aetiological type.

Clinical features

Eyes
Gritty irritation and redness, with early morning stickiness, and reduction in tear secretion (often not noticed by the patient) are the usual features. The dryness may lead to conjunctivitis (Fig. 25), keratitis, corneal erosions and even vascularisation of the cornea.

G-I tract
The salivary glands are usually normal in size but may be enlarged (Fig. 26). Diminished salivary flow is associated with dryness, smoothness and increased sensitivity of the lips and tongue, and dental caries are accelerated (Fig. 27).

Other features
Include respiratory infections, renal tubular defects, atrophic vaginitis, lymphomata.

Laboratory features

Diagnosis established by positive Schirmer's test (measurement of tear secretion with filter paper strip), Rose Bengal and slit lamp examinations (to reveal corneal disease). Biopsy of salivary or lacrimal glands may be necessary to exclude sarcoidosis or malignancy.

Management

Mouth: glycerine mouth wash and sucking lemon sweets.
Eyes: protection and instillation of artificial tears.

Fig. 25 Sjögren's syndrome. Bilateral conjunctivitis in a patient with dry eyes.

Fig. 27 Sjögren's syndrome. Severe dental caries and gingivitis.

Fig. 26 Sjögren's syndrome. Parotid gland hypertrophy. Note scars from duct surgery and biopsy.

3 | Felty's Syndrome

Definition

A syndrome comprising chronic arthritis, splenomegaly and granulocytopenia, named after A.R. Felty (b.1895) in which the lymphoreticular features of rheumatoid arthritis assume an exaggerated form.

Prevalence

Precise prevalence not known. Affects about 1% of patients with rheumatoid arthritis. Splenomegaly alone more common (about 6.5%). F : M; 2 : 1. Onset after at least 10 yr of rheumatoid arthritis. Usual age 50–70 yr.

Aetiology

Variant of seropositive rheumatoid arthritis (see section 1).

Clinical features

1. Severe joint disease (Fig. 28).
2. Splenomegaly (Fig. 28). This is often massive.
3. Hepatomegaly (Fig. 28). Usually slight.
4. Leg ulcers (Fig. 29).
5. Pigmentation—especially legs (Fig. 29).
6. Increased susceptibility to infection.

Radiological features

As under rheumatoid arthritis. Severe destructive arthritis. Abdominal X-ray may reveal splenomegaly.

Laboratory features

Relative and absolute granulocytopenia. Mild to moderate anaemia (most patients). Thrombocytopenia (38%). Rheumatoid factor positive 98%. Positive ANF and LE cells. Anti-DNA not raised.

Management

Aim to reverse haematological abnormalities:
1. Splenectomy if significant morbidity.
2. Drugs have been tried: include corticosteroids, gold, penicillamine, high-dose testosterone (but not for females), and lithium salts.

Fig. 28 Felty's syndrome. Severe, rheumatoid-pattern arthritis with hepato-splenomegaly.

Fig. 29 Felty's syndrome. Severe leg ulcers with pigmentation. Note also arthritis of feet.

Definition

A chronic inflammatory disease of the spine and sacro-iliac joints causing progressive restriction of spinal movement, associated with radiological calcification of spinal ligaments.

Synonyms

Spondylitis ankylopoetica; spondylitis rhizomélique; von Bechterew's disease; morbus Bechterew–Marie–Strumpell.

Prevalence

Established disease: approx. 0.1%. M : F; 5 : 1. Age of onset usually 15–30 yr. Racial variation: less common in American Negroes and more common in American Indians than in Caucasians.

Aetiology

Probably due to a combination of genetic and environmental factors. Genetic transmission is not clear and both Mendelian dominant and multifactorial mechanisms have been reported. Environmental factors could involve infective agents (e.g. *Klebsiella*) and other factors such as trauma.

Clinical features

Spine
1. Pain—worsening at night, and stiffness most noticeable in the morning on wakening.
2. Postural changes may be noted by patient, or only brought to their attention by others. This characteristically involves rounding of the shoulders and slight dorsal kyphosis—the 'hang-dog posture' seen early on (Fig. 30). Later the stoop may become more pronounced (Fig. 31), and in extreme cases limits forward vision.
3. Spinal motion in forward flexion (Fig. 32) and in other directions becomes limited, as does chest expansion.

Peripheral joints
The 'root' joints (hips and shoulders) are most commonly affected (40%). Of other peripheral joint, the knees are most often involved (Fig. 33).

Fig. 30 Ankylosing spondylitis. Early postural changes—the 'hang-dog posture'.

Fig. 31 Ankylosing spondylitis. Advanced stoop with limited forward vision.

Fig. 32 Ankylosing spondylitis. Limited spinal flexion (in patient asked to touch toes).

Fig. 33 Ankylosing spondylitis. Active arthritis of knee with wasted quadriceps.

Radiological features

Pelvis

The crucial radiological feature concerns sacro-iliitis, the presence of which is a sine qua non for diagnosing the disease by international agreement. The components of radiological sacroilitis are:

1. Sclerosis of the margins of the sacro-iliac joint.
2. Blurring of the joint outline due to sacral and iliac erosions.
3. Narrowing and eventually fusion (ankylosis).

The pelvic X-ray is invaluable as, in addition to showing sacro-iliac arthritis (Fig. 34), it may show other features such as symphyseal arthritis, ischial and iliac exostoses, and hip arthritis.

Spine

The most characteristic lesion is the syndesmophyte, the basis of bony bridging. Fig. 35 shows the various stages in the development of intervertebral ankylosis. Other characteristic spinal changes include: vertebral 'squaring', erosion of anterior vertebral corners (Romanus lesions), and disc calcification/ossification. Any region of the spine may be affected but the thoraco-lumbar junction is the best place to look for early changes.

Fig. 34 Ankylosing spondylitis. Bilateral sacro-iliitis and symphyseal arthritis.

Fig. 35 Ankylosing spondylitis. Various stages of intervertebral ankylosis by syndesmophytes.

Co-diseases

1. Iritis (25%). Often unilateral (Fig. 36).
2. Aortic incompetence (1%) (Fig. 37) and, more commonly, cardiac conduction defects.

Less commonly:

3. Cauda equina syndrome (Fig. 38).
4. Atlanto-axial subluxation or spinal fracture.
5. Apical pulmonary fibrosis (resembling tuberculosis).
6. Amyloidosis.

Whether classed as co-diseases, complications, or 'overlap' features, patients with spondylitis may display manifestations characteristic of other spondarthritides: psoriasis, chronic inflammatory bowel disorders, genito-urinary disease.

Laboratory features

ESR raised in 80%, but may be normal even in quite active disease. Often mild anaemia. Test for rheumtoid factor negative. HLA B27 present in 96%.

Management

1. Analgesic/anti-inflammatory drugs (phenylbutazone and indomethacin particularly helpful).
2. Exercises to maintain mobility and prevent development of poor posture.
3. Steroid injection of peripheral joints.
4. Surgery. Hip replacement most often. Only rarely is spinal osteotomy needed, and even then only in special centres.
5. Radiotherapy becoming obsolete because of risk of post-radiation malignancy.

Fig. 36 Ankylosing spondylitis. Unilateral acute anterior uveitis (iritis).

Fig. 37 Ankylosing spondylitis. Left: cardiomegaly due to aortic incompetence. Right: typical 'bamboo spine' in this patient.

Fig. 38 Ankylosing spondylitis. Cauda equina lesion. Note erosions around spinal canal.

5 | Psoriatic Arthritis (1)

Definition

The association of skin or nail psoriasis with seronegative arthritis affecting peripheral and/or spinal joints.

Prevalence

Psoriasis affects 1–2% of the population. About 7% of psoriatics develop arthritis. Of these about 30% have sacro-iliitis. M : F; 1 : 1 for psoriatic arthritis (about the same as in uncomplicated psoriasis—compare female preponderance in rheumatoid arthritis).

Aetiology

Probably due to a combination of genetic and environmental factors. Heredity probably non-Mendelian. Environmental factors could be multifactorial, including physical and emotional trauma, and infection.

Clinical features: dermatological manifestations

Skin
The typical rash consists of salmon-pink, scaly plaques on extensor surfaces (Fig. 39). Variants of this causing circinate, guttate or even exfoliative patterns.
Of importance is the fact that lesions may be minimal (consisting of only a single spot a few millimeters in diameter), or 'hidden'. The scalp is a favourite location for hidden lesions (Fig. 40), but they may be found under the breasts, in the natal cleft or in the umbilicus.

Nail
Nail dystrophy affects about 80% with the uncomplicated skin condition. Typical changes include pitting (Fig. 41), onycholysis (Fig. 42), and other features such as horizontal ridging, keratosis or discoloration.

Fig. 39 Psoriatic arthritis. Typical rash (psoriasis vulgaris).

Fig. 40 Psoriatic arthritis. Patch of scalp psoriasis hidden by hair.

Fig. 41 Psoriatic arthritis. Nail pitting.

Fig. 42 Psoriatic arthritis. Onycholysis.

Clinical features: rheumatological manifestations

1. The commonest pattern is an asymmetrical oligoarticular arthritis involving scattered knuckle joints—DIPs, PIPs or MCPs. A typical example is shown in Fig. 43. The mildness of this pattern of arthritis may lead to the diagnosis being overlooked.
2. It may appear almost indistinguishable from rheumatoid arthritis.
3. The 'textbook' pattern, less common than (1) and (2), is widespread involvement of DIP joints. Although characteristic, it has been over-emphasized in the past as it is seen in only about 5% of patients with psoriatic arthritis.
4. 'Sausage digits'. They may affect the hands (Fig. 44) or feet (Fig. 45), may be generalised, involving all digits, or localised to one finger or toe. This appearance is due to combined IP arthritis and flexor tenosynovitis.
5. Arthritis mutilans occurs rarely. This may be largely 'erosive', giving rise to 'opera-glass fingers' ('doigts-en-lorgnettes'), or 'ankylosing', giving rise to a rigid, clawed hand.
6. Ankylosing spondylitis (see p. 29).

Fig. 43 Psoriatic arthritis. Typical asymmetrical oligoarticular involvement. Note nail dystrophy.

Fig. 44 Psoriatic arthritis. Severe arthropathy with 'sausage fingers'. Note nail dystrophy.

Fig. 45 Psoriatic arthritis. 'Sausage toes' and early toe deformities. Note nail dystrophy.

Radiological features

Often these are no more than periarticular soft-tissue swelling, small periarticular erosions, or diminution of joint space with minimal or no deformity. Other less common radiological features, some of which are shown in Fig. 46, include:
1. Erosion of terminal phalangeal tufts (acro-osteolysis).
2. 'Whittling' of phalanges, metacarpals, and metatarsals.
3. 'Cupping' of the proximal ends of phalanges. The combination of 'whittling' and 'cupping' may give rise to 'the pencil-in-cup deformity' or 'mushrooming'.
4. Ankylosis of phalanges, metacarpals, and metatarsals.
5. Severe destruction of isolated small joints.
6. Predilection for DIP and PIP joints with relative sparing of MP joints (cf. rheumatoid arthritis).
7. Tendency to involve the feet before the hands, as in Reiter's disease.
8. Relative lack of osteoporosis compared with rheumatoid arthritis.
9. Sacro-iliitis (Figs 47 & 48) and even fully established ankylosing spondylitis of identical or similar-type to that seen in idiopathic ankylosing spondylitis.

Laboratory features

Negative for rheumatoid factor. HLA Cw6 associated with psoriasis, HLA DR7 with peripheral arthritis, HLA DR3 with erosive arthritis, and HLA B27 with sacro-iliitis.

Management

1. Integumentary features managed as in the independent skin disorder.
2. Rheumatic features—peripheral arthritis and/or spondylitis, as in those conditions not associated with psoriasis, with some exceptions: try to avoid corticosteroids avoid antimalarials; meticulous care to avoid postoperative sepsis.

Fig. 46 Psoriatic arthritis. Typical changes. Note phalangeal 'whittling' and 'cupping'.

Fig. 47 Psoriatic arthritis. Early sacro-iliitis/spondylitis.

Fig. 48 Psoriatic arthritis. Late sacro-iliitis/spondylitis.

6 | Reiter's Disease (1)

Definition

The triad of arthritis, non-specific urethritis, and conjunctivitis (named after H. Reiter, 1881–1969).

Prevalence

Complicates about 1.7% of patients with non-specific urethritis and about 0.2% with dysentery. M : F; 20 : 1. Usual age of onset about 20–40 yr.

Aetiology

Probably due to a combination of genetic and environmental factors. The latter being, at least in part, infections causing non-specific urethritis or, less commonly, cystitis, prostatitis (the genital type of Reiter's), dysentery or 'non-specific diarrhoea' (the intestinal type).

Clinical features

Acute stage
1. Urethritis (usual).
2. Conjunctivitis (30%)—see Fig. 49.
3. Circinate balanitis (25%)—see Fig. 50.
4. Keratoderma blenorrhagica (15%)—see Fig. 51.
5. Erythema nodosum.
6. Thrombophlebitis.
7. Keratitis.
8. Rheumatological manifestations (see p. 33).

Late stage
1. Iritis (10%).
2. Cardiac conduction defects and aortic incompetence (rare). ,
3. Rheumatological manifestations (see p.33).
Both the acute and later manifestations may be seen in other spondarthritides. For example, the skin lesions may be indistinguishable from pustular psoriasis and the ocular features indistinguishable from those seen in ankylosing spondylitis or in the enteropathic arthropathies.

Fig. 49 Reiter's disease. Bilateral conjunctivitis.

Fig. 50 Reiter's disease. Circinate balanitis.

Fig. 51 Reiter's disease. Keratoderma blenorrhagica.

Clinical features (contd)

Rheumatological manifestations
In addition to arthritis, patients may develop tenosynovitis, usually affecting the Achilles tendon (Fig. 52). In about the same frequency (20%) plantar fasciitis may occur.

The arthritis
Occurs up to about 4 weeks after infection. Knee (90%) and ankle (75%) commonest pattern (Fig. 53). Feet also often affected (40%). Shoulder, wrist, elbow, hip and spine less often involved (30%). Usually asymmetrical (75%) and polyarticular (90%). May be migratory. The spinal involvement—sacro-iliitis or fully developed ankylosing spondylitis—is in general of the type seen in other spondarthritides, with the exception shown in Fig. 54.

Radiological features

1. Peripheral joints may be eroded or ankylosed, but often the arthritis is non-destructive.
2. 'Fluffy' periosteal new bone formation—calcaneal spurs—and periosteal changes around the wrists, ankles or pelvis.
3. Typical changes of ankylosing spondylitis in sacro-iliac and intervertebral joints.
4. 'Bridge lesions' (Fig. 54) not seen in other spondarthritides.

Laboratory features

Much raised ESR. Rheumatoid factor negative. Patients with sacro-iliitis positive for HLA B27.

Management

May be concomitant infection with gonococcus (50%).
1. Treatment of arthritis and spondylitis along routine lines. (Phenylbutazone particularly helpful.)
2. Treatment of associated features and complications. Worth trying oxytetracycline for genital infection, but response may be disappointing.

Fig. 52 Reiter's disease. Achilles tendinitis involving left ankle.

Fig. 53 Reiter's disease. Asymmetrical lower-limb arthropathy.

Fig. 54 Reiter's disease. Spondylitis with 'bridge lesion' and early sacro-iliitis.

7 | Enteropathic Arthropathies

Definition

Arthropathy associated with ulcerative colitis, Crohn's disease or Whipple's disease.

Ulcerative colitis

About 12% of patients with ulcerative colitis (typical barium features are shown in Fig. 55) develop an arthropathy. This is usually a monarticular acute synovitis, but occasionally polyarticular, most often affecting the knees, closely followed by the ankles. Shoulders, elbows, wrists, and small joints of hands and feet are affected less often. The arthritis is non-erosive. It develops either at the onset of colitis or during its course. 'Parallelism' exists between exacerbations of colitis and joint disease. About 30% have sacro-iliitis, some of whom have typical ankylosing spondylitis. Associated features include erythema nodosum, thrombophlebitis, uveitis, and digital clubbing.

Crohn's disease

The typical barium features of Crohn's disease (named after B. C. Crohn, b.1884) are shown in Fig. 56. The features of the arthropathy and the associated features are similar to those described for ulcerative colitis and affect mainly lower limb joints (Fig. 57). (The figure also shows the severe emaciation that may occur from malabsorption.) Sacro-iliitis and spondylitis occur with roughly the same frequency as in colitis, and the features are the same (Fig. 58).

Whipple's disease

Named after G. H. Whipple (1878–1976), and sometimes termed intestinal lipodystrophy, this is a much rarer disease than ulcerative colitis or Crohn's disease. It may be associated with peripheral and spinal arthritis of the type described above.

Fig. 55 Ulcerative colitis. Barium enema showing 'featureless' colon.

Fig. 56 Crohn's disease. Barium follow-through showing the 'string' sign of terminal ileitis.

Fig. 57 Crohn's disease. Emaciation. Synovitis left ankle.

Fig. 58 Crohn's disease. Sacro-iliitis and thoracolumbar syndesmophytes.

8 | Behçet's Syndrome

Definition

A disorder also known as Behçet's disease (after H. Behçet, 1889–1948), the triple symptom complex, or the cutaneo-muco-uveal syndrome, comprising the simultaneous or successive occurrence of genital ulceration, oral ulceration, and uveitis or iridocyclitis.

Prevalence

Rare. Probably more common on Mediterranean littoral and in Japan. M : F; 2 : 1. Peak onset in third decade.

Aetiology

Not known. Some believe it is related to the spondarthritides, some to the vasculitides. Familial in 30%.

Clinical features

Rheumatic manifestations
Inflammatory lower limb arthropathy affecting knees most often (75%) and ankles. Monarticular in 10%. May be migratory.

Asociated features
Aphthous ulcers (100%); genital ulcers (75%); uveitis (75%) (Fig. 59); skin lesions—erythema nodosum (Fig. 60), skin (particular scrotal) ulceration (Fig. 61), sepsis (useful test based on puncture of skin which produces a pustule); thrombo-phlebitis or thrombosis (25%). CNS manifestations (10%); gastro-intestinal (G-I) manifestations (50%); pulmonary lesions.

Radiological features

Peripheral joints normal. Disagreement regarding sacro-iliitis.

Laboratory features

Raised ESR; leucocytosis, hyperglobulinaemia; rheumatoid factor negative; increased HLA B5; biopsy may show vasculitis.

Management

1. Symptomatic.
2. Try corticosteroids and/or immunosuppressives for severe ocular or CNS disease.
3. Avoid needle puncture if possible.

Fig. 59 Behçet's syndrome. Acute anterior uveitis.

Fig. 60 Behçet's syndrome. Erythema nodosum.

Fig. 61 Behçet's syndrome. Scrotal ulcers.

9 | Systemic Lupus Erythematosus (SLE) (1)

Definition

A disorder associated with multisystem involvement and characterised by the presence of antinuclear factor and other auto-antibodies.

Prevalence

Relatively common (probably about 0.5 per 1 000). More common in women (F : M; 9 : 1) and American negroes. Peak age: 20–40 yr.

Aetiology

As with the other systemic connective tissue diseases to be described, the aetiology is unknown. Immunological factors are prominent and there is strong evidence that immune complexes are filtered out of the circulation and are deposited in the basement membrane of the kidney and at other sites affected by the disease.

Clinical features

Joint involvement
Occurs in over 90% cases. Varies in presentation from flitting arthralgia to arthropathy similar to rheumatoid arthritis (Fig. 62). Progressive erosive changes are rare. Aseptic necrosis may occur.

Skin involvement
Sometimes this is a cutaneous vasculitis with overlap features of the type seen in systemic sclerosis or dermatomyositis. In the fingers a typical combination is telangiectasia of the base of the nail (Fig. 63) with digital erythema. The erythema is often more generalised (Fig. 64), affecting the hands, face and other parts. The most characteristic appearance is the 'butterfly' distribution of erythema on the cheeks and across the bridge of the nose (Fig. 64).

Fig. 62 SLE. Rheumatoid-pattern arthropathy.

Fig. 63 SLE. Prominent nailfold capillaries.

Fig. 64 SLE. Typical erythematous rash.

Clinical features (contd)

Skin involvement (contd)
Fig. 65 shows this rash in another patient in further detail. Alopecia (Fig. 66), photosensitivity, Raynaud's phenomenon, and subcutaneous nodules may also be seen.

Involvement of other systems
Renal disease (65%): proteinuria, nephrotic syndrome, and renal failure. Lymphadenopathy (45%). Hepatomegaly (40%). Splenomegaly (25%). Pleurisy with or without effusion (40%). Pericarditis with or without tamponade (25%) (see Fig. 67), and cardiac murmurs. Retinal cytoid bodies (10%) (see Fig. 68). CNS manifestations (fits, psychoses, stroke, chorea) and peripheral neuropathy.

Radiological features

Joints usually normal. X-ray manifestations of associated features.

Laboratory features

Tests to identify circulating auto-antibodies directed against nuclear antigens (LE cell test; fluorescent antinuclear antibody, ANA; DNA-antibody tests—by immunochemical or immunofluorescent means).
Other tests: tests for other auto-antibodies and serum complement level. ESR raised. Immunoglobulins raised. Leucopenia. Skin biopsy examined by fluorescent techniques (immunoglobulin and complement deposition at dermo-epidermal junction).

Management

Corticosteroids are the mainstay of treatment. Antimalarials or an immunosuppressive agent (e.g. azathioprine) may be necessary. Treatment of associated disorders.

Fig. 65 SLE. Typical 'butterfly' rash.

Fig. 66 SLE. Alopecia.

Fig. 67 SLE. Scar from surgical relief of pericardial tamponade.

Fig. 68 SLE. 'Cytoid bodies' (exudates).

10 | Progressive Systematic Sclerosis (Scleroderma) (1)

Definition

A multisystem disorder characterised mainly by inflammation of subcutaneous connective tissue, followed by progressive fibrosis leading to atrophy of skin, subcutaneous fat and associated tissues, and arteritis of skin vessels.

Prevalence

Rare (about 9 per 100 000 females; 5 per 100 000 males). Peak age: 30–50 yr.

Aetiology

Unknown, but strong clinical and serological overlap with other connective tissue disorders.

Clinical features

A typical clinical progression is for a young to middle-aged woman to develop Raynaud's syndrome, followed by hardening of the skin of the fingers and mild arthritis of the knuckle joints. These features may be followed by involvement of internal organs such as the oesophagus. Further clinical details can be summarised thus:

1. *Arthritis.* Mild synovitis of finger joints resembling early rheumatoid arthritis. Combined with oedema of the skin and flexor tenosynovitis, the fingers may assume a sausage shape.
2. *Skin changes.* Vary from mild thickening and induration of the finger tips (acrosclerosis, sclerodactyly) to more widespread involvement affecting arms, upper trunk and face. Telangiectasia commonly accompanies the skin changes (Figs 69, 70 & 71). In addition to telangiectasia, the facies become characteristic with a generalised 'pinched' look, microstomia and fissures radiating from the mouth (Fig. 72).

Fig. 69 Scleroderma. Facies in early disease. A few telangiectases on cheeks and neck.

Fig. 70 Scleroderma. Prominent telangiectasia. 'Steroid facies'.

Fig. 71 Scleroderma. Detail of telangiectatic 'spider'.

Fig. 72 Scleroderma. Facies in advanced disease. Note circum-oral puckering and 'pinches' appearance.

Clinical features (contd)

The appearance of the hands also becomes characteristic due to hardening and thickening of the skin which produce a taut marble-like appearance, with loss of skin creases and clawing (Fig. 73). Other skin features include pigmentation and ulceration of finger tips, knuckles or lower legs. Skin ulceration is associated with subcutaneous calcification in which subcuticular calcific nodules may discharge through the skin (Fig. 74).

3. *Visceral changes.* These include: Raynaud's phenomenon (common); dysphagia (65%), malabsorption or hepatic fibrosis; renal endarteritis with renal failure (20%); Sjögren's syndrome (6%); and rarely fibrosing alveolitis, myocardial fibrosis, pericarditis and other cardiac defects.

Radiological features

1. Resorption of distal phalanges (Fig. 75).
2. Subcutaneous calcification (Fig. 75).
3. Evidence of joint disease—joint space narrowing, periarticular osteoporsis, but no erosions.
4. Barium swallow will show œsophageal changes.

Laboratory features

Modest rise in ESR and in serum globulins. Positive rheumotoid factor in 30%. Most patients have positive fluorescent antinuclear antibody tests.

Management

No really effective treatment available. Advice fc Raynaud's phenomenon. Analgesic/anti-inflammatory drugs for synovitis. Systemic complications will require their own management.

Fig. 73 Scleroderma. Sclerodactyly. Note 'creaseless', clawed and slightly swollen fingers.

Fig. 74 Scleroderma. Calcinosis cutis.

Fig. 75 Scleroderma. Acro-osteolysis with calcific deposits.

11 | Polyarteritis Nodosa

Definition

A disorder in which widespread focal panarteritis with fibrinoid necrosis of the vessel wall produces multisystem disease—particularly affecting the kidneys, heart and nerves.

Prevalence

Rare (exact prevalence not known but <1 : 3500). M : F; 4 : 1. Rare under age 20, or over age 65 yr.

Aetiology

Unknown but evidence for an immunological disturbance, with deposition of immune complexes in vessel walls.

Clinical features

A serious disease with widespread clinical manifestations.
'Rheumatological': generalised muscle/joint pains (70%); arthritis (25%). This may be acute (resembling rheumatic fever) or chronic (resembling RA). Hypertrophic osteoarthropathy may also occur.
Other features: systemic disturbance (fever, weight loss, malaise); renal disease (90%); peripheral neuropathy (50%); cardiovascular hypertension (50%); heart failure or acute pericarditis (30%); painless myocardial infarction (common); lung involvement (30%); skin lesions (25%), including purpura, bruising, livedo reticularis (Fig. 76), dermal infarction (Fig. 77), or more extensive gangrene (Fig. 78); G-I involvement; CNS disease.

Radiological features

In chronic forms, joint changes as in RA. Selective renal angiography may show arterial aneurysms.

Laboratory features

Raised ESR. Neutrophil leucocytosis. Absolute eosinophilia (especially with lung involvement). Mild anaemia. Hypergammaglobulinaemia. Rheumatoid factor positive in 30%. Biopsy of clinically involved tissues positive in about 40%. Characteristic features (Fig. 79) include arterial fibrinoid necrosis and inflammatory cells.

Management

Corticosteroids and immunosuppressive drugs (e.g. azathioprine), but response may be poor.

RHEUMATOLOGY

Fig. 76 Polyarteritis nodosa. Livedo reticularis on elbow region.

Fig. 77 Polyarteritis nodosa. Dermal infarcts on toes.

Fig. 78 Polyarteritis nodosa. Gangrene of toes.

Fig. 79 Polyarteritis nodosa. Biopsy showing widespread fibrinoid necrosis and inflammatory cells.

12 | Polymyositis and Dermatomyositis

Definition

Polymyositis refers to acquire inflammatory disorders of voluntary muscles; proximal weakness being the main feature. When this is associated with skin involvement the term *dermatomyositis* is used.

Prevalence

Rare. F:M; 3:1.

Aetiology

An immunological disturbance. The relationship with virus infection and triggering by malignant disease is still not clear.

Clinical features

The clinical presentation may be divided into childhood and adult dermatomyositis. The latter generally develops in the mid-adult years and may be further divided into:
1. Pure polymyositis. Voluntary muscle weakness affecting mainly proximal limb and girdle muscles.
2. Polymyositis with features of other connective tissue diseases.
3. Other connective tissue disorders with incidental polymyositis.
4. Mixed connective tissue disease—'overlap syndromes', e.g. polymyositis + systemic lupus erythematosus + systemic sclerosis.
5. Adult dermatomyositis (Figs 80–82).

Radiological features

Joints normal. Calcification of skin and proximal limb muscles.

Laboratory features

ESR raised (50%). Raised muscle enzymes (75%)—creatine kinase and aldolase most specific for diagnosis and useful for monitoring treatment. Typical muscle biopsy in 75%. EMG usually abnormal but not specific. Rheumatoid factor positive 50%. ANF positive in 30%.

Management

1. Corticosteroids—if no response one of the remission-inducing agents (e.g. gold, penicillamine, antimalarials).
2. Physiotherapy to improve muscle function.

RHEUMATOLOGY

Fig. 80 Dermatomyositis. Erythema on knees.

Fig. 81 Dermatomyositis. Periorbital heliotrope rash.

Fig. 82 Dermatomyositis. Scaly rash on elbow and forearm.

13 | Osteoarthrosis (1)

Definition

Osteoarthrosis (Syn. osteoarthritis, OA), is a degenerative disease of synovial joints, commonly associated with minor inflammatory features, due to a primary cartilage disorder.

Prevalence

Very common, affecting about 20% of the population. F : M; 2 : 1. Peak onset: age 50 yr. About 50% of the population have radiological changes of OA but only half of these have symptoms.

Aetiolbgy

Not known. Genetic factors probably important in some types. The cartilage disturbance leads to (1) roughening ('fibrillation') and wearing (thinning) of the cartilage surface (leading to exposure of underlying bone); (2) impairment of the cushioning 'shock-absorber' function (leading to damage of underlying bone).

Clinical features

Joints affected: knees 75%, hands 60%— commonest. In the hands, involvement of the DIP joints and carpometacarpal joints gives rise to typical features (Fig. 83). The DIP joint swellings— Heberden's nodes (after W. Heberden, 1710– 1801) are pathognomic and are shown in more detail in Fig. 84. Swellings involving PIP joint are called Bouchard's nodes. The feet are involved in 40%; usually the 1st MTP joint. Hips (25%), ankles (20%), shoulders (15%), and lumbar (30%) and cervical spine (20%) are also affected. When involvement affects a less usual site, in the absence of OA elsewhere, secondary OA should be considered as in Fig. 85.

Fig. 83 OA. DIP joint deformities and hand 'squaring' (carpometacarpal arthritis of thumbs).

Fig. 84 OA. Heberden's nodes.

Fig. 85 OA. Bony prominence over tarsal joints due to secondary osteoarthrosis.

Clinical features
(contd)

Symptoms: pain worse towards evening and aggravated by particular activities. Characteristically, immobility or inactivity stiffness ('gelling'), but morning stiffness may be present.

Signs: bony swelling, soft swelling if effusion present, crepitus, painful limitation of movement, deformity. Baker's cysts or other synovial cysts (e.g. suprapatellar) may occur.

Course: slowly progressive with exacerbations and remissions. Greatest problems arise from involement of weight-bearing joints. No systemic features.

Radiological features

1. Loss of joint space.
2. Sclerosis of adjacent bone.
3. Osteophytes.
4. Subarticular cysts.

These changes can be seen in various joints in the accompanying figures—thumbs (Fig. 86), big toe (Fig. 87), knee (Fig. 88) and hip (Fig. 89). Sometimes articular calcification is an associated feature, and occasionally erosions or ankylosis are present ('erosive OA') but this may be a different disease.

Laboratory

No diagnostic tests.

Management

As for chronic arthritis generally:
1. Analgesic or analgesic/anti-inflammatory drugs.
2. Physiotherapy.
3. Aids and appliances.
4. Surgery.

Fig. 86 OA. Involvement of IP joints of thumb.

Fig. 87 OA. Involvement of 1st MTP joints, left more than right.

Fig. 88 OA. Involvement of tibio-femoral and patello-femoral joints.

Fig. 89 OA. Hip joint involvement (osteophytes, cysts, sclerosis, and joint-space narrowing).

14 | Spondylosis

Definition
Essentially a radiological concept, it refers to all degenerative changes in the spine. Some restrict the term to degenerative changes involving intervertebral as opposed to facetal (synovial) joints (the latter being classed under 'osteoarthrosis').

Prevalence
Very common (see p. 57).

Aetiology
Often follows disc prolapse but aetiology not clear (see p. 57).

Clinical features
Chronic pain, slight stiffness, and root symptoms (see p. 57). In the neck, vertebral artery compression and spinal canal stenosis may occur. Spinal stenosis may also occur in the lumbar region and cause 'neurogenic claudication' due to ischaemia of the cauda equina.

Radiological features
Features identical with osteoarthrosis, notably osteophytes and joint space narrowing. The osteophytes are beak-like (Figs 90–93), may be fused and, when marked, give the spine a gnarled appearance. They must be distinguished from the bony outgrowths of ankylosing spondylitis (these are slimmer and more vertical) and those of ankylosing hyperostosis (these are more exuberant and can involve the entire height of vertebral bodies and not just their marginal lips).

Laboratory features
Unhelpful.

Management
See p. 57 for general principles. Surgical relief may be required for relief of cord compression or osteophyte encroachment on a nerve root.

Fig. 90 Spondylosis. Cervical osteophytes and disc space narrowing. (Lateral view.)

Fig. 91 Spondylosis. Narrowing of cervical intervertebral foramina. (Oblique view.)

Fig. 92 Spondylosis. Lumbar osteophytes. (Lateral view.)

Fig. 93 Spondylosis. Massive lumbar osteophytes with disc space loss and scoliosis. (AP view.)

15 | Disc Lesions

Definition

Cover a wide range from acute disc protrusion in younger patients, to shrinkage of multiple discs and secondary bony overgrowth in older patients.

Prevalence

Very common, increases with age. After age 60 it is rare to find a completely normal spine on X-ray.

Aetiology

In acute cases the annulus fibrosus tears, allowing the nucleus pulposus to herniate. Later, the water content of the disc decreases and it shrinks. Genetic and occupational factors are probably involved.

Clinical features

Acute disc protrusion causes local pain, root symptoms and sometimes signs, limited spinal bending, and scoliosis (Fig. 94). Disc shrinkage and bony overgrowth may also cause local pain and root problems. The commonest spinal segments affected are the lower cervical and lower lumbar regions. The former gives rise to neck pain and 'brachialgia', and the latter to 'lumbago' and 'sciatica'. Rarely, central (as opposed to postero-lateral) protrusion occurs, causing cord compression in the cervical region and cauda equina entrapment in the lumbar region

Radiological features

Plain X-ray: reduced disc space with or without secondary bony overgrowth. Vertical herniations appear as Schmorl's nodes. *Myelography*: indentation of Myodil column (Fig. 95). *Discography:* degenerate disc (normal has central bilobed nucleus).

Laboratory features

Unhelpful.

Management

Cervical and lumbar disc problems: pain relief; rest in bed with or without collar or corset, with or without traction (Fig. 96) in acute phase; preventative advice; mobilisation exercises in post-acute phase; chymopain injection of lumbar discs still controversial; surgery (e.g. lumbar laminectomy) (Fig. 97) only in selected cases.

Fig. 94 Acute lumbar disc lesion. Scoliosis.

Fig. 95 Acute lumbar disc lesion. Myelogram showing identation of Myodil column.

Fig. 96 Acute lumbar disc lesion. Details of leg traction apparatus.

Fig. 97 Acute lumbar disc lesion. Site and extent of healing laminectomy scar.

Definition and aetiology

A disease with a marked familial tendency, occurring mainly in adult men. Characterised by episodes of acute arthritis, and later also by chronic arthritis and damage to soft tissues and kidney. It is caused essentially by hyperuricaemia—an excess of urate in the blood and tissues.

Prevalence

Affects 3–4 per 1 000 (about the same frequency as ankylosing spondylitis). More prevalent in upper social classes, Polynesian races and alcohol drinkers. Affects men after puberty and women after the menopause.

Clinical features

Acute arthritis: affects big toe (MTP joint) in 75% of attacks (Fig. 98). Occasionally ankle, other toes, knee or finger (Fig. 99). Sometimes affects more than one joint (Fig. 100) but monarticular in 90%. Exquisitely painful joint which is red, hot, swollen and very tender. Skin peeling occurs after acute attack. Fever common in acute attacks. Untreated acute attacks last for a few days or weeks, and recur at irregular intervals, sometimes many years apart. Between attacks joints are normal. Later the arthritis becomes chronic and is associated with deformity and tophaceous deposits (Fig. 101).

Fig. 98 Gout. Acute arthritis: dusky, shiny erythema overlying swollen 1st MTP joint.

Fig. 99 Gout. Acute arthritis: erythema and swelling of 3rd PIP joint.

Fig. 100 Gout. Acute arthritis: multiple joint involvement of left foot and ankle.

Fig. 101 Gout. Chronic arthritis: joint deformities associated with massive tophi.

Clinical features (contd)

20% have tophi, characteristically in the helix of the pinna (Fig. 102). Other sites—olecranon and prepatellar bursae, and tendons. Tophi may ulcerate and exude chalky urate salts (Fig. 103). The surrounding inflammation and discharging material may suggest an infected joint, as in the patient shown in Fig. 103.

Associated clinical conditions: obesity (50%); hypertension (50%), vascular disease, and renal failure; renal uric acid stones.

Variants: secondary gout (e.g. myeloproliferative disorders during treatment of malignant disease); renal failure (e.g. lead poisoning—saturnine gout, hyperparathyroidism, hypothyroidism); Lesch–Nyhan syndrome (inherited disorder of urate metabolism); glycogen storage disease.

Radiological features

'Punched-out' radiolucent areas around joints in which there are tophaceous deposits (Fig. 104).

Laboratory features

1. Synovial fluid and tophi contain needle-shaped crystals (Fig. 105). These are strongly negatively birefringent under polarised light.
2. Serum uric acid usually greater than 0.36 mmol/l (6 mg%). Wise to do a series of values.
3. Raised ESR and leucocytosis in acute phase.

Management

Acute attacks: full dosage of indomethacin or other non-steroidal anti-inflammatory drug (e.g. naproxen). Long-term therapy with urate-lowering drugs (uricosurics or allopurinol) may be needed.

Indications: frequent attacks; serum uric acid >0.54 mmol/l (9 mg%); tophi; renal stones.

Fig. 102 Gout. Tophi in classical site on helix of ear.

Fig. 103 Gout. Ulcerating tophus associated with chronic gouty arthritis of 2nd DIP joint.

Fig. 104 Gout. Typical 'punched out' erosions of 1st MTP joint due to tophaceous deposits.

Fig. 105 Gout. Needle-shaped uric acid crystals.

17 | Pseudogout

Definition

A condition otherwise known as pyrophosphate arthropathy associated with deposition of crystals of calcium pyrophosphate dihydrate into joints. The term chondrocalcinosis (a typical feature of pseudogout) should be reserved for the radiological appearance of linear calcification of articular cartilage.

Prevalence

M=F. Age 30+ yr, typically over 60 yr. Earlier onset in familial cases. In elderly patients a 7–28% frequency of meniscal calcification has been reported.

Aetiology

Less is known about the aetiology and pathogenesis of pseudogout than urate gout, but there are similarities between the two diseases in respect of familial tendency, provoking factors, and pattern of disease expression.

Clinical features

Clinical patterns of arthritis are as follows: pseudogout; pseudorheumatoid arthritis; pseudo-osteoarthrosis; pseudo-osteoarthritis with superimposed acute attacks; asymptomatic pyrophosphate deposits; pseudoneurotrophic joints.
The knee is the commonest joint to be affected and the acute features resemble gout. The chronic features resemble OA.

Radiological features

Linear calcification of cartilage (Figs 106 & 107) and degenerative changes indistinguishable from OA.

Laboratory

Synovial fluid: brick-shaped crystals (Fig. 108) which are weakly positively birefringent under polarised light.
Blood: raised ESR and leucocytosis in acute attacks.

Management

Acute stage: aspiration and injection with steroid; analgesic/anti-inflammatory drugs; rest.
Chronic stage: as for osteoarthrosis.

RHEUMATOLOGY

Fig. 106 Pseudogout. Chondrocalcinosis of knee joint articular cartilage.

Fig. 107 Pseudogout. Chondrocalcinosis of hip joint articular cartilage.

Fig. 108 Pseudogout. Rhomboidal crystals of calcium pyrophosphate (grown *in vitro*).

18 | Septic (Suppurative) Arthritis

Definition

Infection of a joint with pyogenic (pus-forming) bacteria.

Prevalence

M : F, 2 : 1. Particularly children and the elderly.

Aetiology

The commonest organism is *Staphylococcus aureus* (50%); *Streptococcocus pyogenes, Str. faecalis, Str. Viridans, E. coli, Haemophilus influenzae, Proteus, Pseudomonas aeruginosa, Klebsiella, Aerobacter, Vibrio fetus* and *Serratia* may cause the same clinical picture. Rarely a complication of infection elsewhere. Usually (70%) a predisposing factor (e.g. RA, diabetes mellitus, joint paracentesis or surgery, steroid therapy, debilitating disease).

Clinical features

Knee most commonly affected (50%). Sometimes other joints (see Fig. 109). Monarticular in 90%. Pain severe. Joint very tender, warm, red and swollen. Fever usual.

Radiological features

Osteoporosis appears after about 2 wk. Thereafter destructive changes may progress rapidly (Fig. 110). Leucocytosis in 90%.

Laboratory features

Macroscopically joint aspiration (or drainage via a scalpel incision) reveals thick yellow-green pus (Fig. 111). Synovial fluid WBC $> 30\,000 \times 10^9$/dl. 90% neutrophils. Gram stain positive in 50%. Culture positive in 85%. If negative repeat for anaerobic culture.

Management

1. Appropriate antibiotic (oral or i.m.).
2. Rest.
3. Daily aspiration.
4. Physiotherapy to restore joint function.

Fig. 109 Septic arthritis. Pus exuding from infected PIP joint.

Fig. 110 Septic arthritis. Large rapidly developing erosions of femoral condyles.

Fig. 111 Septic arthritis. Pus drained from infected knee joint and related calf cyst.

19 | Gonococcal Arthritis

Definition and aetiology

Arthritis due to infection of joints with *Neisseria gonorrhoeae*.

Prevalence

Becoming more common. F:M; 4:1. Any age but particularly young adults. Male patients often homosexual. 0.2% of those with gonococcal urethritis develop arthritis.

Clinical features

Useful points in favour of gonococcal polyarthritis, as opposed to Reiter's disease, are:
1. Patient often female.
2. Upper, as well as lower, limb joints involved.
3. Often involvement of 'unusual' joints (e.g. superior tibio-fibular joint).
4. Characteristic pustular skin lesions.
5. Response to antibiotics.
In view of importance of rash in diagnosis several Figs showing this are included (Figs 112–115). The rash occurs in 70% of patients with arthritis and may be maculopapular, haemorrhagic, vesicular or pustular (as here), particularly in the limbs.

Radiological features

Normal in acute stage. Erosive changes may occur later.

Laboratory

Synovial fluid culture (positive in 50%). Organism may also be recovered from blood, genital tract, anus or pharynx.

Management

1. Penicillin. If hypersensitive or resistant try tetracycline.
2. Counselling and examination of contacts.

Fig. 112 Gonococcal arthritis. Small pustule on finger.

Fig. 113 Gonococcal arthritis. Larger pustule on finger—note erythematous base.

Fig. 114 Gonococcal arthritis. Crop of healing pustules on buttocks and thighs.

Fig. 115 Gonococcal arthritis. Isolated pustule on dorsum of hand.

20 | Tuberculous Arthritis

Definition

Infection of joint or spine with *Mycobacterium tuberculosis.*

Prevalence

Now rare in UK. M > F. Any age, commoner in children and elderly, particularly if debilitated or malnourished.

Aetiology

Joint involvement is usually secondary to involvement of bone. Rarely, direct involvement of synovium occurs.

Clinical features

Joints affected: spine, particularly dorsal region (40%) and hip (25%) commonest sites. May also affect knee (15%), ankle or foot (5%), and sacro-iliac joint (5%).
Insidious onset. Pain minimal at first and often worse at end of day. If untreated, progresses rapidly to deformity and joint destruction. Discharging sinuses may develop.

Radiological features

Typical radiological changes associated with tuberculous peripheral arthritis are (Figs 116–119):
1. Early: normal or osteoporosis.
2. Later: diminished joint space.
3. Erosions and rarely subarticular cysts with sclerotic margins.
4. Smudgy irregular bone outline from destructive changes.
5. Soft-tissue calcification in the healing phase.
The spine shows typically: narrowing of intervertebral space due to disc destruction; areas of osteoporosis and later destructive changes in adjacent vertebrae.

Laboratory

Bacterial confirmation by direct examination, culture and guinea-pig inoculation using synovial fluid or biopsy material.

Management

Chemotherapy as for TB elsewhere; rest; traction or splintage; surgical debridement.

Fig. 116 Tuberculous arthritis. Involvement of hip with soft-tissue calcification.

Fig. 117 Tuberculous arthritis. Long-standing right hip arthritis. Note hypoplasia.

Fig. 118 Tuberculous arthritis. Involvement of elbow, tarsus and metatarsus.

Fig. 119 Tuberculous arthritis. Involvement of tarsus and metatarsus—note calcification.

Hypertrophic Osteoarthropathy/Digital Clubbing/Periostitis (1)

Hypertrophic arthropathy

The syndrome of digital clubbing, painful tender swelling of bones and joints (commonly the ankles and wrists), and radiological periostitis form the characteristic presentation. It may be due to:

1. Benign or malignant, primary or secondary tumours of lung, pleura, heart, diaphragm, mediastinum, or upper G-I tract.
2. Pulmonary suppuration (bronchiectasis, lung abscess, empyema).
3. Aortic aneurysm.
4. G-I disorder (ulcerative colitis, Crohn's disease, steatorrhoea, hepatic cirrhosis).
5. Cyanotic congenital heart disease.
6. An autosomal dominant disorder (rare).

Digital clubbing

Digital clubbing is an essential feature of hypertrophic osteoarthropathy (most commonly seen in middle-aged men with bronchial carcinoma) but also occurs in:

1. Pachydermoperiostosis (Touraine–Solente–Gole syndrome), a syndrome characterised by absence of other underlying disease, periostosis leading to enlargement of the extremities, thickening of the skin and scalp (pachydermia), and an arthropathy.
2. Thyroid acropachy (see under Hyperthyroidism, p. 83).

Clinical features are shown in Fig. 120, with further detail shown in Fig. 121. Apart from soft-tissue swelling of the terminal portions of the fingers (sometimes marked enough to justify the term 'drum-sticking') the nails are curved longitudinally and horizontally, and the angle between nail plate and base of nail is obliterated.

Fig. 120 Digital clubbing. Note all fingers affected.

Fig. 121 Digital clubbing. Detail: nail curvature and obliterated nail plate/nail bed angle.

Hypertrophic Osteoarthropathy/Digital Clubbing/Periostitis (2)

Periostitis

Definition

Periostitis (or periosteitis, but not periostosis) is a term to describe radiographic periosteal shadowing due to new bone deposition and calcification outside the bone cortex.

Types

1. 'Onion-skin appearance'—periosteal new bone formed in layers with translucent tissue between them (e.g. secondary deposit from neuroblastoma).
2. 'Sun-ray appearance'—subperiosteal calcification formed at right angles to the bone shaft (e.g. osteosarcoma).
3. Narrow linear shadow running more or less parallel to the cortex (Figs 122–125). This is the most common appearance (e.g. periostitis of hypertrophic osteoarthropathy).

Causes

The causes of periosteal shadowing include: post-traumatic shadowing; non-traumatic haematoma; stress, fatigue or pseudofracture; inflammatory conditions (e.g. pyogenic, syphilitic, tuberculous, or fungal infections of bone); benign neoplasms (e.g. osteoid osteoma); malignant neoplasms (e.g. Ewing's tumour); vascular disorders (varicose veins, arterial occlusion); hypertrophic osteoarthropathy (see p. 71); pachydermoperiostosis; melorheostosis.

Fig. 122 Periostitis. Early involvement of phalanges and metacarpals. Radius and ulna also affected.

Fig. 123 Periostitis. Marked involvement of forearm bones, particularly radii.

Fig. 124 Periostitis. Involvement of both femora.

Fig. 125 Periostitis. Marked involvement of tibiae and fibulae. Femora also affected.

Carcinoma arthritis

Definition

A rheumatic disorder clinically resembling RA, occurring in any type of malignant disease (particularly in carcinoma of the bronchus, prostate and breast), but not due to metastases in bone or joint.

Prevalence

M : F; 2 : 1. Peak age 50–65 yr.

Aetiology

Unknown. Mechanisms based on alterations of cellular immunity or circulating immune complexes have been suggested, but remain unproven.

Clinical features

Carcinoma arthritis may be the presenting feature of malignancy. In others, clinical features relating to a specific malignant condition will be present. Common examples of such features are shown in Figs 126–128.
1. Onset typically about 1 yr before manifestation of malignancy.
2. Joints affected: knees, ankles, MCP and MTP joints commonest; 20% monarticular; 50% asymmetrical; joints may be warm, red, swollen, and tender in acute stage.
3. Course: variable, usually remits with control of malignancy.

Radiological features

Usually normal.

Laboratory features

Non-specific blood and synovial evidence of inflammation.

Management

1. Control of associated malignant disease.
2. Analgesic/anti-inflammatory drugs.

Fig. 126 Carcinoma arthritis. Underlying cause—bronchogenic carcinoma right lung.

Fig. 127 Carcinoma arthritis. Underlying cause—prostatic carcinoma. Note gynaecomastia from stilboestral therapy.

Fig. 128 Carcinoma arthritis. Underlying cause—pancreatic carcinoma presenting with jaundice.

Metastases

Definition

The term metastasis (Gr. a removing = *meta* + *stasis* = a placing) in reference to cancer denotes the appearance of neoplasms in parts remote from the primary tumour.

Clinical and radiological features

The clinico-radiological implications of skeletal metastases (most often from a bronchogenic carcinoma) in rheumatology are as follows:

1. Pain from single or multiple metastases, often evident as osteolytic or osteosclerotic lesions on X-ray (Figs 129–132) may initially be ascribed to 'fibrositis' or other forms of soft-tissue rheumatism.
2. Polyarthritis may result from metastatic invasion of joints. Usually asymmetrical.
3. Symmetrical metastatic finger deposits may resemble RA. Picture may be additionally confusing if patients are seropositive for rheumatoid factor (20% with malignancy seropositive).
4. Phalangeal metastases may simulate gout, osteomyelitis or tenosynovitis by direct synovial implantation or by involvement of juxta-articular bone.
5. Involvement of the axial skeleton may mimic spondylosis with or without radiculopathy.

Management

1. Treatment of rheumatic manifestations. Symptomatically with analgesics or analgesic/anti-inflammatory drugs. Narcotic analgesics may be required.
2. Treatment of the primary (if known) and secondary deposits if possible with chemotherapy and/or radiotherapy according to clinical circumstances.

Fig. 129 Metastases. Multiple, discrete osteoblastic secondaries in ribs and scapulae.

Fig. 130 Metastases. Multiple, discrete osteoblastic secondaries throughout pelvis.

Fig. 131 Metastases. Patchy sclerosis due to secondaries in vertebrae.

Fig. 132 Metastases. Isolated secondary in acromion—an unusual site.

Myelomatosis

Definition

Chronic, progressive, invariably fatal disorder due to malignant plasma cell proliferation characterised by the development of multiple bone tumours.

Prevalence

M : F; 2 : 1. Peak age 50–70 yr.

Aetiology

Unknown.

Clinical features

Bone pain occurs in 90%. Pain is localised to the joints in 15%. Three types of arthritis occur:
1. Due to myeloma deposits in bone near joints.
2. Associated with amyloidosis.
3. Arthritis resembling carcinoma arthritis.
Additional rheumatic effects may arise from pathological fractures, nervous system involvement, chronic renal insufficiency and the effects of corticosteroids.

Radiological features

A classical X-ray finding is the 'pepper-pot' skull (Figs 133 & 134) due to osteolytic deposits. Similar deposits may occur near joints and in the pelvis. Osteoporosis is seen particularly in the spine and may, together with lytic lesions, cause vertebral collapse. Pathological fractures may also be revealed on X-ray.

Laboratory features

ESR usually >50 mm/h. Paraprotein on electrophoresis in 75%; diminished immunoglobulin levels. Bence–Jones proteinuria in 40%. Hypercalcaemia in 50%. Bone-marrow aspiration reveals plasma-cell infiltration—confirmatory.

Management

Radiotherapy to painful areas; analgesic/anti-inflammatories, and narcotics later if necessary.

Fig. 133 Myelomatosis. 'Pepper-pot skull' showing multiple lytic deposits—lateral view.

Fig. 134 Myelomatosis. 'Pepper-pot' skull—anteroposterior (AP) view.

Pituitary gigantism/acromegaly

Definition

Pituitary adenomas causing chronic over-production of growth hormone cause gigantism before, and acromegaly after, epiphyseal closure.

Prevalence

F : M; 3 : 2. Commonest age of acromegaly onset: 20–40 yr. 50% of acromegalics have arthropathy.

Aetiology

Pituitary adenoma causes increased anabolism (mainly of collagen) and cellular proliferation (mainly fibroblastic).

Clinical features

1. Before epiphyses close, gigantism due mainly to increased 'longitudinal' growth occurs. May be associated with aches and pains, and postural changes, but no clear-cut rheumatic syndromes.
2. After epiphyseal closure, longitudinal growth no longer being possible, 'horizontal' growth occurs, seen as gradual enlargement of the bones and soft tissues of the head (Figs 135 & 136), hands (Fig. 137), and feet. Main rheumatic features of acromegaly are: low backache; limb arthropathy (often knees); entrapment neuropathies (usually carpal tunnel syndrome); neuromuscular symptoms; Raynaud's phenomenon.

Radiological features

Tufting of distal phalanges; increased joint space; exostoses–phalangeal 'lips' and 'hooks' and spinal osteophytes; calcification of joint capsule and cartilage; thickened, widely-spaced trabeculae; enlarged pituitary fossa.

Laboratory features

Insulin and glucose-tolerance tests, and growth hormone level confirmatory.

Management

1. Treatment of adenoma (hypophysectomy), but this has no effect on arthropathy.
2. Analgesics.
3. Carpal tunnel decompression.

Fig. 135 Acromegaly. Typical facies in profile.

Fig. 136 Acromegaly. Prognathism —note over-riding lower teeth.

Fig. 137 Acromegaly. Large spade-like hands of patient, compared with a normal hand.

Thyroid

**Hypo-
thyroidism**

Patients with deficiency of thyroid hormone may develop a constellation of rheumatic manifestations. The typical facies (Figs 138 & 139) will often alert diagnostic suspicion, but sometimes general clinical features are more masked. The principal rheumatic syndromes associated with hypothyroidism are:

1. Pain and stiffness in proximal muscles.
2. Polyarthritis. Bilateral and symmetrical. Usually affects knees, often wrists, MCP or MTP joints, and occasionally ankles and elbows. This is an inflammatory arthropathy although there may be superimposed osteoarthrosis.
3. Monarthritis associated with osteolytic lesions, usually in children.
4. Carpal tunnel syndrome.
5. Secondary gout.
6. Pains in neck, shoulders, and upper chest in about 10% of patients with Hashimoto's thyroiditis.

**Hyper-
thyroidism**

Hyperthyroidism (appearance shown in Figs 140 & 141) is not a cause of arthritis, but rheumatic manifestations may occur:

1. Myopathy affecting proximal muscles and associated with weakness and cramp.
2. Thyroid acropachy. This affects about 1% of hyperthyroid patients and is characterised by soft-tissue swelling of fingers and toes, digital clubbing, pretibial myxoedema and exophthalmos. It follows successful treatment of hyperthyroidism.

Fig. 138 Hypothyroidism. Typical myxoedema facies in female patient.

Fig. 139 Hypothyroidism. Less obvious myxoedema facies in male patient.

Fig. 140 Hyperthyroidism. Note goitre. Otherwise appearance normal.

Fig. 141 Hyperthyroidism. Note lean face and bright, slightly prominent eyes. Goitre not obvious.

Adrenal

Addison's disease

A condition due to *hypo*activity of the adrenal cortex (named after T. Addison, 1793–1860). Although not responsible for rheumatic features, its therapy may be. Fig. 142 shows an Addisonian patient treated with corticosteroids which, in excess or on withdrawal, may give rise to musculo-skeletal pain.

Cushing's syndrome

A condition due to *hyper*activity of the adrenal cortex (named after H. Cushing 1869–1939). Identical features may develop to those seen with long-term, high-dose corticosteroid therapy. In addition to the superficial stigmata of the syndrome (Figs 143 & 144), patients may develop the following:

1. Profound osteoporosis, resulting in crush fractures of vertebral bodies with wedging and severe back pain.
2. Avascular necrosis of the femoral or humeral head.
3. Rheumatic manifestation due to 'general' features of the disease (e.g. muscle wasting) and to rheumatic features of 'complications' (e.g. diabetes mellitus).
4. Although poorly documented, it might be expected that inadequate replacement therapy after surgical treatment might give rise to the steroid-withdrawal rheumatic syndrome of intense arthralgia, joint tenderness, and periarticular oedema.

Fig. 142 Addison's disease. Note pigmentation across forehead. Cushingoid facies from steroid therapy.

Fig. 143 Cushing's syndrome. Pre-operative facies in patient with adrenal adenoma.

Fig. 144 Iatrogenic hypercorticism. Striae atrophicae due to steroid therapy for RA.

Syringomyelia

Definition

The presence of cavities (Gr. *syrinx* = tube or pipe) surrounded by gliosis near the central canal of the spinal cord and medulla.

Prevalence

Age of onset: 10–60 yr; usually 25–40 yr, M : F; 3 : 1.

Aetiology

Probably based on a congenital abnormality with abnormal closure of the embryonic spinal canal and secondary gliosis of the cavities thus formed.

Clinical features

Onset very insidious. Wasting and weakness of the small muscles of the hand are the commonest early symptoms. Sensory or trophic lesions may be the first to attract attention. These patients are sometimes referred to rheumatologists in the mistaken belief that the diagnosis is 'arthritis'. The features giving rise to erroneous diagnosis include: finger contractures (Figs 145 & 146); digital mutilation (Fig. 147); limitation of joint motion and power (Fig. 148).

Radiological features

Trophic changes of terminal phalanges may suggest scleroderma, psoriatic arthritis, or polvinyl-chloride disease. Charcot's arthropathy may be present—about 25% having this feature (see p. 89).

Laboratory features

Unhelpful.

Management

1. Irradiation of the affected region of the spinal cord and medulla.
2. Treatment of Charcot's joints (see page 89).
3. Physiotherapy to improve muscle power.
4. Local treatment for trophic skin changes.
5. Avoidance of further trauma.

Fig. 145 Syringomyelia. 'Main en griffe' and cigarette-burn scars.

Fig. 146 Syringomyelia. 'Benediction hand'—note muscle wasting and associated prominent thumb CM joint.

Fig. 147 Syringomyelia. Mutilated, fleshy ('main succulente'), scarred hand.

Fig. 148 Syringomyelia. Weakness and wasting with severely limited abduction.

Charcot's arthropathy

Definition

A condition characterised by marked disorganisation of a joint and destruction of joint surfaces, associated with diminished pain sensation named after J. M. Charcot (1825–93).

Prevalence

Depends on cause but, in general, an uncommon disorder. M : F; 3 : 2. Usually after middle age, but may be seen in children with congenital lesions.

Aetiology

Most common predisposing disorders are: tabes dorsalis; diabetes mellitus; syringomyelia. Rarer causes include: hereditary sensory radicular neuropathy and Charcot–Marie–Tooth disease; congenital indifference to pain; spinal cord disease and peripheral nerve lesions; familial dysautonomia.

Clinical features

Pain may be present initially, but is often absent or diminished in later stages. Monarticular in 70%—often the knee. *Acute stage*: warm, tender, swollen joint. *Chronic stage*: swelling, instability, crepitus and grotesque deformity (Figs. 149 & 150).

Radiological features

Sclerosis of bone ends; realignment and remodelling; loss of joint space; loose bodies; massive osteophytes; periarticular calcification; fractures. Most of these features are shown in Fig. 151.

Laboratory features

Unhelpful.

Management

Rest in acute stage. Avoidance of traumå. Later: stabilisation with appliances to prevent or correct deformity. Consider arthrodesis, but bear in mind that non-union may occur.

Fig. 149 Charcot's arthropathy. Charcot knee with secondary arthritis of ankle and foot.

Fig. 150 Charcot's arthropathy. Detail of above. Note deformity and marks from supporting bandage.

Fig. 151 Charcot's arthropathy. Gross destruction, degenerati[ve] bodies (AP and lateral views).

Carpal tunnel syndrome

Caused by compression of the median nerve at the wrist, it is the most common of the 'entrapment neuropathies'. It occurs in adults of all ages, particularly in women. It may be idiopathic or associated with various general disorders, e.g. obesity, pregnancy, myxoedema, acromegaly, rheumatoid arthritis and osteoarthrosis. The features of pain and muscle wasting may be mistaken for the results of joint disease, as may the relative prominence of wrist and thumb bones due to muscle wasting (Fig. 152).

Herpes zoster

Infection of the posterior root ganglion with the varicella virus, causing segmental pain and a vesicular rash (Fig. 153), may be associated with two types of rheumatic disorder:
1. Arthritis of the small joints of the hand in the distribution of affected nerves.
2. Shoulder–hand syndrome. The painful pre-rash stage may suggest arthritis of peripheral or spinal joints.

Polyneuropathy

This is of rheumatological relevance for two reasons:
1. If due to a purely neurological disorder the symptoms (pain, paraesthesiae) and signs (motor and/or sensory deficit) may suggest a rheumatic disorder.
2. It may be an established complication of a chronic rheumatic disorder (e.g. RA, SLE). Clinical signs, such as the one shown in Fig. 154, will clarify the significance of the neuropathy; in this case toxic polyneuropathy due to lead poisoning manifested by the classical blue line on the gums.

Fig. 152 Carpal tunnel syndrome. Right thenar wasting with prominence of CM joint.

Fig. 153 Herpes zoster. Eruption localised to right T9 dermatome.

Fig. 154 Lead poisoning. Typical blue line at upper and lower gingival margins.

Neuralgic amyotrophy

A condition characterised by pain in the shoulder, which may be mistaken for the shoulder—hand syndrome or frozen shoulder. More common in men (M : F; 2 : 1). History of preceding illness, operation, or trauma in 50%. Main features: sudden pain in shoulder, followed by limited movement and, later, nerve palsy. The neurological deficit, most often serratus anterior paralysis (Fig. 155), recovers slowly over 12—18 mth and does not recur.
Treatment: analgesics and physiotherapy.

Neurofibromatosis

This hereditary disease (von Recklinghausen's disease, after F. D. von Recklinghausen 1833—1910) is characterised by multiple neuromas or neurofibromas (Fig. 156), pigmented skin lesions and neurological manifestations due to involvement of nerve trunks, nerve roots and spinal cord. Skeletal manifestations include kyphoscoliosis, hyperostosis of facial bones, enlargement of the calvarium, and hyperostosis and curvature of long bones.

Intracranial tumour

As with stroke syndromes, this may enter into rheumatological differential diagnosis (Fig. 157). Cerebral changes may be confused with antirheumatic drug effects or the psychological and psychiatric manifestations of systemic rheumatoses (e.g. SLE); weakness and deformity in limbs may be ascribed to concomitant arthritis, particularly in the elderly.

Fig. 155 Neuralgic amyotrophy. Winging of right scapula due to paralysis of serratus anterior.

Fig. 156 Neurofibromatosis. Plexiform neuroma affecting right eye and cutaneous fibromata.

Fig. 157 Intracranial tumour.

Haemorrhagic disorders

The main rheumatological impact of haemorrhagic and related disorders is blood in the joint—haemarthrosis. This may occur in various conditions, including primary synovial sarcomata, pigmented villonodular synovitis, osteoarthrosis, rheumatoid arthritis, pseudogout, after trauma, as well as in primary haematological disorders (notably haemophilia). The physical signs of a hot, tender joint with or without surface manifestations of peri-articular haematoma are similar whatever the cause. The patient shown in Fig. 158 had RA, but the appearance would be similar in haemophilia. Scurvy has been included here (Fig. 159) as massive ecchymoses may occur (particularly in adults) near joints but not in them. (These patients may also develop arthritis.)

Haemoglo- binopathies

Certain haemoglobinopathies, particularly sickle-cell disease, may be associated with rheumatological features. In sickle-cell disease it is the homozygotes who develop arthritis due to bone infarcts resulting from thrombotic crises. This also occurs in sickle-cell and β thalassaemia, in addition to the typical clinical (Fig. 160) and laboratory features of haemoglobinopathies. The main radiological signs are: areas of porosis or sclerosis representing infarcts; dactylitis due to periosteal proliferation; evidence of bone marrow hyperplasia in the skull ('hair-on-end' appearance), spine ('cupped' vertebrae, Fig. 161), and long bones near joints (cortical thinning and widening of medulla); avascular necrosis; salmonella osteomyelitis.

Fig. 158 Haemorrhagic disorders. Haemarthrosis with peri-articular haematoma in RA.

Fig. 159 Haemorrhagic disorders. Massive ecchymosis due to scurvy.

Fig. 160 Haemoglobinopathies. Leg scars in sickle-cell disease.

Fig. 161 Haemoglobinopathies. Spondylopathy in sickle-cell disease. Note cupped vertebrae.

26 | Diseases of the Digestive System

Upper G-I tract

Conditions of rheumatological significance are: aphthous ulcers (e.g. Behçet's syndrome, ulcerative colitis); oesophagitis (e.g. drug therapy); peptic symptoms or ulceration (e.g. drugs (Fig. 162), underlying neoplasia); chronic inflammatory small bowel disease (e.g. Crohn's disease, Whipple's disease); malabsorption due to rheumatoid-induced amyloidosis; infarction due to RA.

Lower G-I tract

Conditions of rheumatological significance are: ulcerative colitis (Fig. 163); Crohn's colitis; Behçet's syndrome; Reiter's disease; shigellosis; colonic and rectal neoplasms.

Liver

Liver disease (often little more than altered liver function, without histological changes) is seen in RA and its variants (e.g. Felty's syndrome and Sjögren's syndrome). SLE may be associated with occasional perihepatitis. Unrelated to SLE, chronic active hepatitis with LE cells ('lupoid hepatitis') may be associated with an arthritis simulating RA. Hepatic involvement may be a prominent feature in certain malignant disorders (Fig. 164) which may have rheumatic accompaniments.

Pancreas

Acute pancreatitis, chronic relapsing pancreatitis and pancreatic carcinoma may be associated with transient polyarthritis, accompanied by tender nodular skin lesions due to subcutaneous fat necrosis. The arthritis is usually synchronous with the skin lesions but may precede them, and other manifestations of pancreatic disease, by several weeks. Apart from biochemical tests, the plain abdominal X-ray may give valuable clues concerning the presence of pancreatic disease. Note pancreatic calcification in Fig. 165.

RHEUMATOLOGY

Fig. 162 Upper G-I tract. Barium meal showing gastric ulcer, probably steroid-induced.

Fig. 163 Lower G-I tract. Barium enema showing colitis on left (right normal).

Fig. 164 Liver disease. Hepatosplenomegaly. (This patient had Hodgkin's disease.)

Fig. 165 Pancreatic disease. Pancreatic calcification in chronic active pancreatitis.

Diseases of the Urinary System

General comment

Diseases of the urinary system, principally of the kidneys, may be associated with a multitude of rheumatic ailments. The renal–rheumatic association may occur as part of a systemic connective tissue disorder (e.g. SLE), as part of a nephrotoxic syndrome (e.g. analgesic nephropathy), or as the musculoskeletal manifestations of chronic renal failure, dialysis, or transplantation.

Clinical features

The musculoskeletal features of renal disease include the following: secondary hyperparathyroidism; osteomalacia; calcium pyrophosphate arthropathy (pseudogout); extraskeletal calcification; acute gouty arthritis; monarticular, crystal-negative arthritis; polyarticular, crystal-negative arthritis; septic arthritis.
Apart from osteoarticular manifestations, the usual general stigmata of acute and chronic renal disease should be sought. Naked-eye examination of the urine is an integral part of the clinical examination (Figs 166 & 167).

Radiological features

These may be divided into those relevant to osteoarticular manifestations (covered elsewhere in this book under appropriate sections), and those concerning examination of the urinary tract. The value of the plain abdominal X-ray (Fig. 168) should not be underrated, although more detailed examination by means of contrast radiography (Fig. 169) will be necessary in most patients.

Management

This is according to the specific nature of the osteoarticular problem (see appropriate section) and the type of urinary tract problem.

Fig. 166 Renal disease. Facies of a patient in chronic renal failure.

Fig. 167 Renal disease. Haematuria.

Fig. 168 Plain radiograph. Can provide useful information. Kidney on right is normal.

Fig. 169 IVP. Duplex kidney and ureter (with hydronephrosis) on left.

28 | Hypercholesterolaemia

Definition

An hereditary disorder of cholesterol metabolism characterised in homozygotes by a markedly raised plasma cholesterol, xanthomatosis and premature atherosclerosis. It may be associated with arthritis.

Prevalence

Rare. M = F. Onset 5–10 yr.

Aetiology

Autosomal intermediate transmission.

Clinical features

50% of homozygotes develop arthritis. The characteristics of this are: acute onset, often migratory, affecting large joints—usually knees. Cholesterol deposits present as unilateral (Fig. 170) or bilateral (Fig. 171) xanthelasma. Xanthomata at other sites, e.g. elbows (Fig. 172) and in relation to tendons and periosteum. Other features include: corneal arcus, premature atherosclerosis, and cardiac murmurs.

Radiological features

Joints usually normal. May be phalangeal erosions not involving joint surface.

Laboratory features

Raised plasma cholesterol. ESR raised in attacks of arthritis.

Management

Symptomatic: salicylates.
Diet: low cholesterol and high polyunsaturated fat diet. Cholestyramine.

RHEUMATOLOGY

Fig. 170 Hypercholesterolaemia. Unilateral xanthelasma palpebrarum.

Fig. 171 Hypercholesterolaemia. Bilateral xanthelasma palpebrarum.

Fig. 172 Hypercholesterolaemia. Xanthomata on elbow.

29 | Sarcoidosis

Definition

A condition of unknown aetiology characterised by multisystem involvement due to granulomatous inflammation particularly affecting lymph nodes, spleen, liver and lungs. There may be an associated arthritis and the details below concern this (as opposed to the parent disorder).

Prevalence

F : M; 3 : 1. Age 15–50 yr; peak 20–30 yr. Affects about 10% of patients with sarcoidosis.

Aetiology

Both the cause and mechanism of this disease are unknown but many theories have been proposed, mainly based on hypersensitivity.

Clinical features

Arthritis of sarcoidosis of two types:
1. Early acute transient type. This often affects wrists (Fig. 173), elbows (Fig. 174), shoulders, MCP and PIP joints. Rarely big toe— resembling gout.
2. Chronic persistent type.

Radiological features

Joints usually normal. Cystic changes occasionally seen in hands or feet. Chest X-ray shows hilar lymphadenopathy (Fig. 175) in 75% and/or pulmonary infiltration (50%).

Laboratory features

Raised ESR, tests for rheumatoid factor positive in 10%. Hypergammaglobulinaemia (10%). Mantoux negative in 70%. Kveim test positive in 70%. Synovial biopsy or biopsy of other tissues— granulomata and inflammatory changes.

Management

Analgesic/anti-inflammatory drugs. Steroids for severe 'resistant' arthritis or for other indications (e.g. iritis, hypercalcaemia).

Fig. 173 Sarcoidosis. Acute arthritis of wrist. Note shiny erythema overlying joint.

Fig. 174 Sarcoidosis. Acute arthritis is elbow and erythema nodosum on forearm.

Fig. 175 Sarcoidosis. Bilateral hilar lymphadenopathy.

30 | Toxic Erythemas

Erythema nodosum

An acute self-limiting disorder characterised by an eruption consisting of painful and tender nodules in the skin on the front of the legs (Fig. 176) and back of the forearms (Fig. 177). The lesions are at first bright red, later darker, and eventually fade like bruises. The acute illness may be accompanied by malaise, fever, and joint pain and swelling (note arthrocentesis site Fig. 176). Associated conditions include: sarcoidosis (commonest cause in UK—35% of all cases); various infections, particularly streptococcosis and primary tuberculosis; ulcerative colitis, Crohn's disease, Behçet's syndrome; malignant disease; drug sensitivities, e.g. to sulphonamides; idiopathic—10%.
Treatment: rest + aspirin or other NSAIDs.

Erythema multiforme

An eruption consisting of circular or irregular erythematous blotches. These are often 'target' or 'iris' lesions (Fig. 178). The rash commonly occurs on the backs of hands and forearms. Polyarthritis is an uncommon complication. It often follows drug therapy or vaccination. Often no cause is found. No specific treatment available. Antibiotics may be needed to control secondary infection of eye or mucosal lesions. Systemic steroids may be required for severe bullous or mucosal types.

Other erythemas

Erythema marginatum has been mentioned under rheumatic fever. Generalised erythema having scarlatiform, morbilliform, macular or circinate features may be associated with drug therapy, other dermatoses, or infections (e.g. syphilis), all of which may be accompanied directly or indirectly by joint involvement.

Fig. 176 Erythema nodosum. Rash on both legs and synovitis of knees (right joint aspirated).

Fig. 177 Erythema nodosum. Rash on both forearms. Site infrequent but appearance of lesions typical.

Fig. 178 Erythema multiforme. Typical 'target' lesions.

31 | Osteoporosis

Definition	Osteoporotic bone is normal in composition but reduced in amount—skeletal atrophy or osteopenia.
Prevalence	Depends on cause. Commonest types are post-menopausal and 'senile' osteoporosis.
Aetiology	*Idiopathic*: post-menopausal, 'senile' (or elderly), pregnancy, young adult, juvenile. *Known or postulated*: immobilisation, endocrine, chromosomal (Turner's syndrome), with osteomalacia, other (including RA, osteogenesis imperfecta).
Clinical features	Localised pain, deformity, fracture. The commonest deformity is loss of height due to vertebral collapse ('shrinkage' in old people is due to osteoporosis). Examination may reveal loss of trunk height, a transverse abdominal crease (Fig. 179A) and kyphosis (Fig. 179B).
Radiological features	Before structural collapse, porotic changes become evident (Fig. 180—normal spine, *left*, and porotic spine, *right*). Vertical trabeculae become more prominent due to loss of horizontal trabeculae. Irregular wedging of vertebrae (Fig. 181), without the prominent 'cod-fish spine', due to vertebral concavity seen in osteomalacia (except in the young or in inherited osteoporosis).
Laboratory features	Plasma and urine values within normal range. Biopsy sometimes done to exclude other disorders (e.g. osteomalacia, leukaemia, myeloma).
Management	*Prevention*: exercise, avoiding immobility. Mechanical supports (braces). Oral calcium supplements, vitamin D, fluoride, anabolic steroids, calcitonin, parathormone have been tried, but evidence conflicting. Most convincing treatment is oestrogen therapy in post-menopausal women.

RHEUMATOLOGY

Fig. 179A

Fig. 179B

Fig. 180

Fig. 181

32 | Osteomalacia and Rickets

Definition

Difficult to define. There is defective mineralisation of organic bone matrix, seen histologically in undecalcified bone as an excess of osteoid. Rickets is the childhood disorder; osteomalacia the adult counterpart.

Prevalence

Depends on cause. Becoming more prevalent in UK since increase in Asian population.

Aetiology

Causes are: vitamin D deficiency; malabsorption; renal disease; other disorders (e.g. anticonvulsant osteomalacia, tumour rickets, vitamin D-dependent rickets).

Clinical features

Main symptoms are bone pain, deformity, tenderness, and weakness of proximal muscles. Deformity is most marked during childhood (bowing of long bones, 'rickety rosary', Harrison's sulcus, and bossing of frontal and parietal bones). Clinical features from underlying disorder (e.g. renal failure, malabsorption).

Radiological features

In rickets the characteristic features are widening of the growth plate and of the metaphysis, which is cupped and ragged. In osteomalacia the classical sign is the Looser's zone (after E. Looser 1877–1936). This is the radiological hallmark of active osteomalacia and appears as a ribbon-like area of demineralisation (Fig. 182: pelvic Looser's zones; Fig. 183: Looser's zones in forearm bones). The vertebral bodies are porotic and uniformly biconcave (Fig. 184A: 'cod-fish' spine). When parathyroid activity is prominent the 'rugger-jersey' spine (Fig. 184B) may be a feature due to increased density of end plates.

Laboratory features

Histology (see above); total plasma calcium low or normal; inorganic phosphate low; alkaline phosphatase usually increased. Urinary calcium low. Urinary phosphate increased.

Management

Vitamin D. Treatment of underlying disorder.

RHEUMATOLOGY

Fig. 182

Fig. 183

Fig. 184A

Fig. 184B

33 | Paget's Disease of Bone

Definition

A disorder of unknown aetiology (named after J. Paget 1814–99) affecting one or more bones, particularly the pelvis, femur, skull, tibia and vertebrae.

Prevalence

Rare before age 30 yr; 0.5% at 40 yr; 10% at 90 yr. M : F; 2 : 1. In the UK about 650 000 have Paget's disease (but only 5% with symptoms).

Aetiology

Cause not known but pathophysiology is characterised by disorganised overactivity of bone, with parallel activities of rapid resorption and rapid laying down of new bone.

Clinical features

Mainly bone pain and deformities. Four types of arthritis may occur: arthritis due to disease adjacent to joint; calcific periarthritis; acute gout; spondylopathy simulating spondylitis. Characteristic features include large skull (Fig. 185), bowed tibia (Fig. 186), deafness, kyphosis. Rarer features: spinal cord, nerve root or cauda equina compression, high output cardiac failure, and osteogenic sarcoma.

Radiological features

Typical features of this 'busy-bone' disorder are shown in Fig. 187. Note the 'fluffy' appearance of the bone, coarse trabeculation and expansion and thickening of affected bones. The disease does not cross joint lines.

Laboratory features

Alkaline phosphatase usually raised. Plasma calcium usually normal, plasma phosphate may be in upper normal range. Urinary total hydroxyproline increased. Bone biopsy required only rarely to confirm diagnosis or exclude malignant disease.

Management

Analgesics; 'specific' treatment with calcitonin, mithramycin or EHDP; treatment of complications (e.g. fractures, cardiac failure, osteogenic sarcoma).

RHEUMATOLOGY

Fig. 185 Paget's disease. Enlarged skull.

Fig. 186 Paget's disease. Mid-shaft bowing of tibia ('sabre tibia').

Fig. 187 Paget's disease. Typical changes. Note hip joint line not crossed.

Definition

Excessive formation of parathormone usually by an autonomous parathyroid adenoma (rarely hyperplasia or carcinoma).

Prevalence

Present in 3–10% of patients with recurrent renal calculi. F : M; 5 : 1. Age of onset: 30–70 yr.

Aetiology

This can be explained in terms of the main effects of parathormone which are: to reduce re-absorption of phosphate; to stimulate osteoclastic bone resorption; to stimulate renal reabsorption of calcium and calcium absorption across the small intestine.

Clinical features

Arthritis is a rare presenting feature. It may follow parathyroidectomy. The main types of arthritis in this disorder are:
1. Osteogenic synovitis due to softening and collapse of subchondral bone, arthritis occurring for same reason as in osteomalacia.
2. Pseudogout due to hypercalcaemia.
3. Gout due to diminished tubular uric acid secretion.

Non-rheumatological features include:
1. Anorexia, vomiting and constipation.
2. Polyuria, polydypsia and renal colic.
3. Weakness and tiredness.
4. Band keratopathy.
5. Mental changes.

Radiological features

Subperiosteal reabsorption of the phalanges (Fig. 188) is diagnostic. It is thought to occur more markedly on the radial border of the proximal and middle phalanges of the index and middle fingers (Fig. 189). Resorption and shortening may affect the distal phalanges (Figs 188 & 189) but is not pathognomonic (it also occurs in polvinylchloride workers' disease, scleroderma and psoriatic arthritis).

Fig. 188 Hyperparathyroidism. Distribution of subperiosteal erosions and acro-osteolysis.

Fig. 189 Hyperparathyroidism. Further details of subperiosteal erosions and acro-osteolysis.

**Radiological
features**
(contd)

Resorption may also occur in the medial borders of the upper tibiae, symphysis pubis, femoral necks and outer ends of clavicles. Occasionally more localised lesions are seen. These include 'cysts' in the ribs or other bones and a 'pepper-pot' appearance in the skull. Cortical resorption and trabecular coarsening may also give the skull a Paget's-like appearance (Fig. 190). The spine may show the 'rugger-jersey' effect (Fig. 191—see absent but this is of little diagnostic value. Soft-tissue calcification may be present (fig. 191).

**Laboratory
features**

1. Raised serum calcium, low phosphate.
2. Alkaline phosphatase may be increased, but is normal if there is no clinical or radiological evidence of bone disease (the majority).
3. Raised urea in later stages.
4. Hyperuricaemia in 50%.
5. ESR normal.
6. Tests for rheumatoid factor negative.

Management

Orthodox teaching is that the only treatment for primary hyperparathyroidism is surgical. However, conservative management is reasonable for asymptomatic patients with mild hypercalcaemia (> 3 mmol/l). The operation should involve removing the adenoma together with identification and examination of the remaining three glands (10% have multiple adenomata).

Fig. 190 Hyperparathyroidism. Typical features in skull due to cortical resorption and trabecular coarsening.

Fig. 191 Hyperparathyroidism. 'Rugger-jersey spine'. Also note aortic calcification.

**Definition
and
aetiology**

Bone necrosis usually due to interference to the blood supply, which may be due to arteritis, external vascular pressure, trauma, thrombosis or embolism. Clinical subdivisions of avascular necrosis are: traumatic; secondary to existing arthropathies; secondary to systemic conditions; idiopathic.

Prevalence

May occur at any age, in either sex, depending on the underlying cause.

**Clinical
features**

Usually one or both hips. Rarely knees or shoulders. The condition is bilateral in 30%. Features of underlying disease, if there is one.

**Radiological
features**

Examples of early (Fig. 192) and later (Fig. 193) avascular necrosis, due to RA, are shown here. The main radiological stages can be summarised as follows:

1. A crescentic area of rarefaction of subchondral bone.
2. Irregularity or flattening of the affected epiphyses, or a depressed segment of subchondral bone.
3. An area of porosis, or patchy sclerosis, which in the hip joint appears as a sector of the femoral head.
4. Separation of necrotic fragments, particularly in the knee, and collapse of bone underlying the sector of affected joint surface.
5. Complete joint destruction, or disappearance of the femoral or humeral heads.

**Laboratory
features**

Unhelpful.

Management

Best without weight-bearing, sometimes allows healing and remodelling. Surgical treatment with arthroplasty often required when the joint becomes severely deformed.

Fig. 192 Avascular necrosis. Relatively recent destructive changes. Note 'fluffy' irregularity of femoral head.

Fig. 193 Avascular necrosis. Long-standing destructive changes. Note well-defined margin of pseudoar-throsis.

36 Ankylosing Hyperostosis (Forestier's Disease)

Definition

Also known as Zuckergusswirbelsaüle, hyperostotic spondylosis, vertebral melorheostosis, Forestier's or Baastrup's disease. This is a condition of the elderly in which there is exuberant bony outgrowth from the spine.

Prevalence

Most commonly seen in men aged 50+ yr. Frequency: 14% in males and 5% in females over age 35+ yr.

Aetiology

Some regard it as a variant of spondylosis but it is probably a separate entity. It has been attributed to increased growth hormone output, but little is known about its aetiology, and no family surveys have been recorded.

Clinical features

Often asymptomatic. Sometimes stiffness without pain. Examination may reveal slight restriction of spinal movement but this is not of spondylitic pattern. No postural changes. Peripheral joint involvement not a feature. Diabetes mellitus often associated.

Radiological features

Typical patterns of ossification are shown in Fig. 194–196. Characteristically the layer of ossification extends throughout the entire height of some vertebrae (Fig. 196). The ossified protuberances may extend upwards as 'candle-flame' lesions or downward as 'dripping candle-wax'. The apophyseal joints and the sacro-iliac joints (Fig. 197) are normal, distinguishing the disorder from ankylosing spondylitis.

Laboratory features

ESR normal. Calcium, phosphates and alkaline phosphatase normal. HLA B27 negative. Rheumatoid factor negative.

Management

Urine and blood tests may reveal diabetes mellitus symptomatic. Maintenance of mobility.

Fig. 194 Ankylosing hyperostosis. Exuberant flamed-shape exostoses over front of cervical vertebrae.

Fig. 195 Ankylosing hyperostosis. Bamboo-like thoracic spine due to thick bands of paravertebral ossification.

Fig. 196 Ankylosing hyperostosis. 'Candle-wax' (or 'sugar-icing') ossification throughout upper lumbar vertebrae.

Fig. 197 Ankylosing hyperostosis. Pelvic exostoses. Note patency of sacro-iliac joints.

37 | Marfan's Syndrome

Definition

An inherited disorder characterised by skeletal deformity, arachnodactyly, dislocated lenses and aortic dilatation (named after A. B-J. Marfan 1858–1942).

Prevalence

Rare—estimated at 1.5 per 1 000 000 of the population.

Aetiology

Autosomal dominant inheritance with wide variability of expression.

Clinical and radiological features

Excessive lengthening of the digits—arachnodactyly (Fig. 198)—is one of the cardinal features, although it is not pathognomonic. The tall asthenic build and 'El Greco' facies are also characteristic (Fig. 199), although non-asthenic forms do exist. Disproportionately long extremities (Fig. 200), a high palate, thoracic asymmetry, and articular hypermobility are other typical skeletal features. 50% have eye defects; most commonly ectopia lentis. 20% have cardiovascular anomalies, including septal defects, conduction defects and aneurysms. Later manifestations are aortic incompetence and dissecting aneurysm. Backache occurs in 30%, and 20% have peripheral arthritis.

Laboratory features

In the urine, homocystine is absent (cf. homocystinuria which may resemble Marfan's syndrome) and hydroxyproline may be increased.

Management

Treatment of aortic valve disease (the main cause of death). Other features requiring treatment include scoliosis and excessive growth, especially in girls. This has been achieved by an oestrogen–progesterone regime.

Fig. 198 Marfan's syndrome. Arachnodactyly. Note long, thin phalanges and metacarpals.

Fig. 199 Marfan's syndrome. Note 'El Greco' facies, pectus excavatus, 'linear' somatype.

Fig. 200 Marfan's syndrome. Typically, span exceeds height. (Patient also had RA.)

Definition

An hereditary disease caused by a deficiency of the enzyme homogentisic acid oxidase. It is associated with alkaptonuria—the excretion of 'alkaptan', later identified as homogentisic acid, and ochronosis (*ochros* = sallow), the accumulation of pigment in tissues.

Prevalence

Rare. M : F; 2 : 1.

Aetiology

Inheritance by an autosomal recessive character. The lack of homogentisic acid oxidase causes metabolic changes through defective catabolism of phenylalanine and tyrosine.

Clinical features

Degenerative arthritis of peripheral joints—knees (80%), shoulders (50%) and hips (50%). Degenerative spondylopathy. The peripheral arthritis clinically resembles osteoarthrosis, and the spinal changes, spondylosis. However, if limitation of spinal motion and chest expansion is prominent, the spondylopathy may resemble ankylosing spondylitis.

Associated features:

1. Black, dark-brown or bluish discoloration of sclera (Fig. 201), cornea, conjunctiva, eyelids and skin, and ear cartilages (Fig. 202). This usually appears in middle age.
2. Renal and prostatic calculi.
3. Darkening of urine which becomes black on standing or when alkalinised (see p. 125).

RHEUMATOLOGY

Fig. 201 Alkaptonuria. Patches of ochronotic pigment in sclerae.

Fig. 202 Alkaptonuria. Ochronotic pigment in lower part of auricular cartilage.

Radiological features

Spine
Dense calcification of intervertebral discs (Fig. 203) is characteristic, indeed pathognomonic. This is associated later with: narrowing of disc spaces, sclerosis of adjacent vertebral margins, and, ultimately, disappearance of discs and vertebral fusion (Fig. 204). The sacro-iliac joints are normal. There is no ligamentous calcification.

Peripheral joints
Narrowing of joint space with irregularity of joint surface, sclerosis, cystic changes, and osteophytes.

Laboratory features

As mentioned before, the urine darkens on standing (Fig. 205) or on alkalinisation. When fresh, the urine may be a normal colour. It will give a positive reaction when tested for reducing substances, but not with glucose oxidase. This may lead to an erroneous diagnosis of diabetes mellitus from the use of Benedict's test or Clinitest tablets, or to failure to detect reducing substances if glucose oxidase (Clinistix) is used.

Management

Symptomatic treatment with analgesics. The logical approach, to reduce homogentisic acid precursors from the diet (e.g. tyrosine or, less specifically, protein) has met with little success.

Fig. 203 Alkaptonuria. Intense calcification of intervertebral discs—pathognomic for the disease.

Fig. 204 Alkaptonuria. Marked degenerative changes—intervertebral ossification anfd disc space narrowing.

Fig. 205 Alkaptonuria. Progressive darkening of urine on standing.

39 | Pseudoxanthoma Elasticum

Definition

An hereditary disorder caused by a defect in elastic tissue associated with characteristic skin and eye changes, and arterial disease.

Prevalence

Rare. Skin lesions slightly more common in females, angioid streaks more frequent in males.

Aetiology

Autosomal recessive inheritance, with partial limitation to the female found most often. Irregular dominance has been described.

Clinical features

Cutaneous lesions are small, soft chamois-coloured papules parallel to skin lines and folds. This gives rise to a crepe-like or Moroccan leather appearance. Another dermal feature is the 'plucked chicken skin' appearance. Sites most often affected are the side of the neck (Fig. 206), axillae, groins, cubital and popliteal fossae, and the peri-umbilical area. Angioid streaks of the retina are the most characteristic eye lesions and produce the 'tigroid fundus' (Fig. 207). Premature and advanced arterial changes are also common in this disorder. Arthritis is not usually a feature, but intermittent pain, tenderness, and swelling of joints have been reported.

Radiological features

None of rheumatological significance. (Arthropathy is not destructive.)

Laboratory features

Biopsy reveals characteristic features—notably calcification in the middle and lower dermis (Fig. 208).

Management

Symptomatic treatment for cardiovascular disease. Plastic surgery sometimes helpful to correct cosmetic cutaneous defects.

Fig. 206 Pseudoxanthoma elasticum. Typical skin features include the 'plucked chicken skin' appearance side of neck.

Fig. 207 Pseudoxanthoma elasticum. 'Tigroid fundus'. Note broad, pale, angioid streaks around optic disc.

Fig. 208 Pseudoxanthoma elasticum. Calcification in middle and lower dermis.

40 | Hypophosphataemic Spondylopathy

Definition

Familial hypophosphataemia is a variant of renal or vitamin D-resistant rickets. Childhood rickets heals spontaneously at puberty and is replaced later in life by a spondylitis-like picture—hypophosphataemic spondylopathy.

Prevalence

Rare. F : M; 3 : 1.

Aetiology

Inheritance is by an X-linked dominant character.

Clinical features

Often more severe in men. Onset after age 20 yr, sometimes presenting in the elderly. Spine, hips and elbows commonly affected. Often also shoulders, knees, wrists, ankles, hands and feet. Gradual onset of stiffness; morning stiffness slight. Pain minimal.

Radiological features

The radiological changes include ligamentous calcification, new bone formation, and generalised demineralisation of bones. This is particularly prominent in the spine (Figs 209 & 210), in and around the pelvis (Fig. 211), and at ligamentous attachments in relations to large joints such as the shoulder (Fig. 212). Obliteration of the sacro-iliac joints may occur (see Fig. 211), and this may raise the question of ankylosing spondylitis (in which a past history of rickets may be helpful).

Laboratory features

Serum phosphates low. Serum calcium low or normal. Raised alkaline phosphatase. HLA B27 not yet studied.

Management

Symptomatic: drugs for pain and stiffness, and cautious physiotherapy as there may be demineralisation of bones.

Fig. 209 Hypophosphataemic spondylopathy. Ossification of anterior spinal ligaments of cervical spine.

Fig. 210 Hypophosphataemic spondylopathy. Ossification and generalised porosis of lumbar vertebrae.

Fig. 211 Hypophosphataemic spondylopathy. Spondylitis-like ossification of pelvis and hips.

Fig. 212 Hypophosphataemic spondylopathy. Exostoses at muscle attachments around shoulder.

41 | Osteogenesis Imperfecta (Fragilitas Ossium)

Definition

Hereditary disease of bone characterised by recurrent fractures and severe deformities.

Prevalence

One of the most common of the inherited disorders of the skeleton.

Aetiology

Autosomal dominant inheritance, variable in expression. Complete non-penetrance has been reported.

Clinical features

Bone fragility is the cardinal feature. This predisposition is variable, some patients experiencing multiple fractures, others few. The fractures heal rapidly, sometimes with residual deformity. A wide bi-temporal diameter and pearly-grey discoloration of the teeth are variable concomitants. Although also variable, blueness of the sclerae (Fig. 213) is a particularly characteristic and classic feature. Fig. 214 shows the same feature in an asymptomatic relative. Deafness supervenes in adulthood in about 20%.

Radiological features

Fracture(s). Florid callus formation may simulate osteosarcoma. In the 'thick bone' type, the shafts of the long bones are short and wide. In the 'thin bone' type, the diaphyses are gracile. Undermineralisation becomes prominent later in life. The shafts of long bones may become expanded and cystic. The base of the skull may become flattened.

Laboratory features

Not helpful.

Management

Genetic counselling, but the variable expression of the disease can give rise to difficulties.

Fig. 213 Osteogenesis imperfecta. Patient with blue sclerae (right), control (left).

Fig. 214 Osteogenesis imperfecta. Patient's asymptomatic daughter with blue sclerae.

42 | Some Other Metabolic Bone Diseases

Diaphyseal aclasis

This is one of the most common inherited skeletal disorders. Multiple bone swellings appear in infancy and increase in number and size until growth stops. The ends of the long bones (Fig. 215), the pelvis and shoulder girdle are most commonly involved. The lesions may be painful or 'silent'. Infrequently, severe deformity and diminution of stature may develop. The most important complication is malignant degeneration.

Albright's syndrome

Named after F. Albright (b.1900), and also termed polyostotic fibrous dysplasia, this disorder is characterised by widespread and often unilateral bone disease, unilateral pigmentation and (in females) precocious puberty. Thyrotoxicosis, acromegaly, and Cushing's syndrome may also be associated for reasons yet obscure. The commonest form is the monostotic type, often in the upper end of the femur. The cystic bone changes, which vary in shape and size (Fig. 216), may be extensive and progressive in the polyostotic type. The 'shepherd's crook' deformity of the femur (not shown here) is characteristic. Treatment has included calcitonin (with little success) and orthopaedic correction of deformities.

Synovial osteochon-dromatosis

A condition, which is often confused terminologically with osteochondromatosis (previous term for both diaphyseal aclasis and Ollier's disease), associated with the formation of cartilaginous plaques within the synovium. By metaplasia these may ossify (Fig. 217). Clinical problems are associated with effusion, 'locking' and premature OA. Treatment is surgical removal of loose bodies or synovectomy.

Fig. 215 Diaphyseal aclasis. Massive exostoses at muscle attachments of both knee joints.

Fig. 216 Albright's syndrome. Cysts in pelvis and femur. Pseudofracture left femoral neck.

Fig. 217 Synovial osteochondromatosis. Multiple intrasynovial ossified bodies at back of knee joint.

43 | Juvenile Chronic Arthritis (JCA) (1)

Definition

A group of diseases of uncertain aetiology which (by definition) begin before age 16 yr. Variously labelled 'juvenile rheumatoid arthritis' and 'Still's disease' (after G. F. Still, 1868–1941) in the past, but now evident that several distinct syndromes are involved.

Prevalence

Details not yet known, but condition is rare. Probably about 5 000 cases in the UK, i.e. approx. 1 : 10 000. F : M; 1.7–3.2 : 1.

Aetiology

Probably varies according to type of disease, e.g. juvenile RA probably has different aetiology from juvenile spondarthritis. A varying blend of genetic, environmental and immunological factors are likely to be involved.

Clinical and radiological features

Clinical types are as follows:
1. *Systemic.* Onset 1–3 yr. High swinging fever. Lymphadenopathy, hepatosplenomegaly, pericarditis and pleurisy. Seronegative for rheumatoid factor.
2. *Polyarticular seronegative.* Younger girls.
3. *Polyarticular seropositive.* Older girls. Antinuclear factor positive 75%.
4. *Pauci-articular* (2 types).
a. Girls under 5 yr. *Chronic* iridocyclitis affects about 5%.
b. Older boys. Associated with sacro-iliitis, HLA-B27 and *acute* iridocyclitis

Both (a) and (b) seronegative. Other types seen less often. May be associated with psoriasis, Reiter's disease, or inflammatory bowel disease; or one of the collagen disorders. (These may or may not be related to one of the 'established' groups.)

Fig. 218 JCA. Brachydactyly associated with IP and MCP joint arthritis.

Fig. 219 JCA. Radial deviation at PIP joints.

Fig. 220 JCA. Ankylosis and severe deformity with radial deviation (adult).

Juvenile Chronic Arthritis (JCA) (2)

The arthritis: some characteristic clinical features of the hand arthritis are shown on p. 136. Brachydactyly due to metacarpal shortening (Fig. 218), *radial* deviation of fingers (Fig. 219), and ankylosis (Fig. 220) are fairly typical of juvenile, as opposed to adult, rheumatoid arthritis.

In addition to involvement of knuckle joints and wrists (and counterpart joints in the feet), other joints may also be involved. In fact no joint is exempt. The knees are commonly affected: Fig. 221 demonstrates advanced knee arthritis with valgus deformity (probably aggravated by obesity) and Fig. 222 shows severe fixed flexion deformity. (Medical treatment was effective in reducing the latter but not the former.) More often, however, the knee arthritis is no more than a recurring synovitis with effusion, settling over a few years with little residual damage or deformity.

The temporomandibular joints (TMJs) may become arthritic, and dental hygiene may become a problem due to inability to open the mouth sufficiently (Fig. 223). Another repercussion of jaw joint disease is hypoplasia of the mandible. This gives rise to micrognathos, or brachygnathism (receding chin), variously termed bird, shrew or mouse facies (Fig. 224). This appearance has been reported in up to 30% of patients. Other growth disturbances due to inhibition or overgrowth of bones will be mentioned overleaf (see under 'Management').

Fig. 221 JCA. Valgus deformity of knees. Note hands and feet also involved.

Fig. 222 JCA. Fixed flexion deformity of knees.

Fig. 223 JCA. Severe dental caries. TMJ involvement.

Fig. 224 JCA. Micrognathos ('shrew facies') TMJs involved.

Clinical and radiological features (contd)

A characteristic feature of some patients with JCA, suggesting a link with the spondarthritides, is sacro-iliitis and even fully developed ankylosing spondylitis (Fig. 225). Cervical spine involvement (with fusion) may be particularly troublesome. This illustration, which also shows hip joint fusion, serves to emphasise the strong ankylosing diathesis in peripheral as well as in spinal joints in some juvenile patients.

In addition to the non-articular features already mentioned, the rash (Fig. 226) of JCA deserves special mention. This affects about 45% of patients and consists of patches of erythema on the trunk and limbs, often seen towards the end of the day and made prominent by a hot bath. In most patients it is not itchy, but if pruritus is present, it is intense. The rash often shows perimacular blanching ('haloes'), and the Koebner phenomenon may be prominent.

Other associated features, taking JCA as a whole, are fever (20%); splenomegaly (35%); lymphadenopathy (45%); pericarditis (10%); iritis (10%); nodules (5%); and, less commonly, abdominal pain due to mesenteric adenitis or peritonitis, and various CNS effects (drowsiness, irritability, fits, and meningism) in the acute stage.

Laboratory features

See under sub-types (p.135). In addition, leucocytosis common in systemic disease.

Management

General principles—drugs, remedial therapy, surgery—as for adult inflammatory arthritides, with the following exceptions: if rest is required, be watchful for development of joint fusion; regular slit-lamp examination for iritis; ensure continued education; avoid contact sports; when possible *avoid systemic corticosteroids* as these may aggravate the natural tendency of the disease to cause growth stunting (Fig. 227). If necessary use alternate-day steroids or ACTH.

Fig. 225 JCA. Ankylosed sacro-iliac joints, hip arthritis, and symphyseal changes.

Fig. 226 JCA. Macular erythema.

Fig. 227 JCA. Patient with stunted growth (on steroids) standing next to her mother. [Courtesy North-Holland]

44 | Rheumatic Fever and Rheumatic Heart Disease

Definition

An acute febrile illness characterised by arthritis, carditis and chorea that follows streptococcal infection.

Prevalence

Now much less frequent and less severe in UK, but still common in some parts of the world. M=F. Peak age 5–15 yr. Rare below age 3 yr and above 20 yr.

Aetiology

Hypersensivity to group-A haemolytic streptococcus. Lesions probably due to antigen–antibody immune complexes. Predisposing factors include social class (overcrowding), age (children), and slight familial influence.

Clinical features

History of sore throat 1–3 wk before polyarthritis in most patients. The disorder has an acute onset, the main features being arthritis, fever, night sweats, recurrent epistaxis and abdominal pain. The joint disorder is a migratory polyarthritis affecting mainly large joints (knees and ankles commonest). Less commonly other joints may be involved (Fig. 228). Arthritis settles without residua. 40% develop carditis and a proportion ultimately develop chronic heart disease due to valvular scarring (Fig. 229). Subcutaneous nodules occur in 10%, chorea in 10%, and erythema marginatum in 5%.

Radiological features

Joints normal. Chest X-ray shows cardiac and pulmonary features especially in chronic rheumatic heart disease with 'decompensation' (Fig. 230).

Laboratory features

Raised ESR; positive throat swab in 25%; ASO titre raised in 75%; raised LDH with carditis; ECG—conduction defects, signs of pericarditis or myocarditis.

Management

Rest. Aspirin. Penicillin in acute phase. Treatment of cardiac complications. (Note heart surgery scar in Fig. 229.)

RHEUMATOLOGY

Fig. 228 Rheumatic fever. Acute arthritis of wrist joints and scattered PIP joints.

Fig. 229 Chronic rheumatic heart disease. Malar flush, pigmentation, raised JVP, hepatomegaly and cardiac surgery scars.

Fig. 230 Mitral stenosis. Straight left heart border, small aortic knuckle, hilar congestion and Kerley's lines.

Henoch–Schönlein Purpura and Other Childhood Vasculitides

Henoch– Schönlein purpura

Henoch—Schönlein or Schönlein—Henoch purpura is a disorder named after J. L. Schönlein (1793–1864) and E. H. Henoch (1820–1910). The condition is characterised by an exanthem associated with G-I manifestations or arthritis, or both. The condition may follow an upper respiratory tract infection which is often streptococcal. The rash, typically found on the buttocks (Fig. 231), is at first urticarial and itchy. Later muculopapular lesions, changing from pink to deep purple, occur. These gradually fade over about 2 wk. Biopsy of the skin lesions shows characteristic perivascular changes. Arthritis lasts only a few days. Other manifestations tend to last up to 6 wk but resolve completely, except for the renal disorder which may be more prolonged. *Treatment*: salicylates or other NSAIDs. Not steroids.

Other childhood vaculitides

In addition to Henoch–Schönlein purpura there are many other forms of childhood vasculitis, either occurring as primary diseases or secondary to other systemic disorders. Classification is difficult but follows that proposed for adults, with some exceptions. Fig. 232 shows an example of allergic vasculitis which is similar in many respects to Henoch–Schönlein purpura, except that the skin lesions are more varied, more truncal and more prominently urticarial, and G-I involvement is less prominent.

Fig. 231 Henoch–Schönlein purpura. Typical distribution of vasculitic rash.

Fig. 232 Urticarial vasculitis. Urticaria with scratch marks.

Digital Contractures/ Deformities (1)

Shoulder-hand syndrome

This is a painful disability of the shoulder appearing before, during, or after pain, swelling and vasomotor changes in the hands and fingers. It may be associated with finger contractures (Fig. 233), and these may evolve into a Dupuytren's-like appearance. Associated features include: idiopathic onset (25%); myocardial infarction (20%); cervical spondylosis (20%); trauma (10%); hemiplegia (5%); drugs such as phenobarbitone, isoniazid or ethionamide; malignancy (pulmonary or cerebral); any form of shoulder arthritis; herpes zoster.

Dupuytren's contracture

This is a common disorder in which progressive fibrosis of the palmar fascia causes painless flexion contractures of the fingers. It affects men more often than women (8 : 1) and appears after the age of 25 yr. It is occasionally familial, and has a significant association with liver disease, especially alcoholic cirrhosis, and epilepsy. The ring finger is affected first and most prominently, then the little finger, middle finger, index finger and thumb. Puckering of the palmar skin is typical (Fig. 234) and is associated with thickening and sometimes nodules in the palmar fascia. May be associated with knuckle pads or Peyronie's disease. Treated by selective fasciectomy.

Campto-dactyly

Implies flexion contracture of PIP joint, typically of fifth finger (Fig. 235). May be confused with clinodactyly (see p. 147) and this term often used synonymously. It may be familial or sporadic.

Fig. 233 Shoulder–hand syndrome. Note oedema and digital contracture of left hand.

Fig. 234 Dupuytren's contracture. Digital contracture with palmar puckering.

Fig. 235 Camptodactyly. Flexion contracture of both little fingers.

Digital Contractures/ Deformities (2)

Clinodactyly

Denotes a flexion contracture with radial curvature. This usually affects the PIP joints of the fifth finger (Fig. 236). The condition may occur sporadically or as a familial disorder showing dominant inheritance. Like camptodactyly, it is of little clinical consequence.

Syndactyly

This term refers to bone or soft-tissue union of two or more digits. The extent of the anomaly is variable. Syndactyly is a component of several genetic syndromes. It may exist in isolation either as a genetic or non-genetic entity. In general, the genetic forms are bilateral and fairly symmetrical. Fig. 237 shows unilateral (and probably non-genetic) syndactyly.

Polydactyly and poly-syndactyly

The presence of an extra digit is termed polydactyly. If digital fusion is also present the term polysyndactyly is used. It may be genetic or non-genetic. Polydactyly is conventionally classified into pre-axial (duplication of thumb or great toe) and postaxial (duplication next to fifth digit). Fig. 238 is therefore an example of pre-axial polysyndactyly.

Intra-uterine amputation

Intra-uterine amputation by amniotic bands is thought to be a common cause of amelia (incidence 1 in 5 000–10 000 births). Grooves around limbs or evidence of partial amputation provide additional clues for the action of this process. A typical example of intra-uterine amputation is shown in Fig. 239.

Fig. 236 Clinodactyly. Flexion and radial deviation of little finger.

Fig. 237 Syndactyly. Note 'fused' toes and vestigial nail.

Fig. 238 Polysyndactyly. Double thumbs. (Patient also had nodular RA and pseudoaxanthoma elasticum.)

Fig. 239 Intra-uterine amputation. Note smooth stump in otherwise normally proportioned finger.

Digital Swellings

Knuckle pads

Otherwise known as the knuckle-pad syndrome, knobbly knuckles or Garrod's fatty pads. They appear as fleshy pads over the dorsa of PIP joints (Fig. 240) at any age in either sex. Sometimes painful and tender, and may give rise to suspicion of nodular RA. However, the joints are clinically and radiologically normal. Often an associated Dupuytren's contracture. Reassurance is mainstay of therapy.

Neoplastic swellings

Although isolated solid swellings on the fingers are often rheumatoid nodules, Heberden's or Bouchard's nodes, or gouty tophi, occasionally they turn out to be neoplastic. Two examples are shown here (Figs 241 & 242). The ivory osteoma had all the features of a malignant deposit clinically. Remember that renal neoplasms have a particular tendency to metastasise to finger bones.

Cystic swellings

Occasionally Heberden's nodes may appear as cystic swellings. Synovial bulging of PIP joints may also resemble a cyst if localised. The cyst in Fig. 243 was an implantation dermoid. Usually a history of a penetrating injury. Should be excised if causing inconvenience.

Another cystic swelling in the hand is a ganglion. This is a tense thin-walled cyst that develops over a joint capsule or tendon sheath. Firmness to the point of feeling 'bony' is characteristic of flexor tendon ganglia. A very common site is on the dorsum of the wrist. They may subside spontaneously. If painful, surgical removal is the most effective treatment.

Fig. 240 Knuckle pads. Typical fleshy (and painful) swellings, affecting all fingers.

Fig. 241 Synovioma. Biopsy revealed a benign growth.

Fig. 242 Ivory osteoma. This ulcerating metatasis-like growth was benign.

Fig. 243 Implantation dermoid. This cyst appeared without any obvious history of penetrating injury.

Iatrogenic Lesions: Drug Rashes

Non-steroidal anti-inflammatory drugs (NSAIDs)

When a rash occurs in a patient taking NSAIDs (or any antirheumatic drug for that matter) the question of drug eruption arises. The rash may take many forms, and in many instances mimics that due to a non-iatrogenic cause. The main aid to diagnosis (short of rechallenge) is the knowledge that particular reaction patterns are favoured by certain drugs, and that amongst these some are more common offenders than others. Fig. 244 shows aspirin-induced urticaria, the commonest eruption associated with this drug. Other aspirin-induced rashes include angioneurotic oedema, fixed eruptions, erythema multiforme, and purpura.

Cortico-steroids and corticotrophin

Dermatological manifestation of large doses of corticosteroids or corticotrophin are those associated with hyperactivity of the adrenal cortex: cutaneous atrophy with increased skin fragility, bruising, purpura, striae, local pigmentation, acne, hirsutism and superimposed infections (e.g. buccal candidiasis). More generalised pigmentation may occur with corticotrophin. A typical example of 'steroid skin' is shown in Fig. 245—a patient needing long-term corticosteroids for rheumatoid arthritis.

Remission-inducing drugs

Remission-inducing drugs commonly cause rashes. Fig. 246 shows a papular erythema associated with penicillamine. Other skin problems due to this drug include purpura, lichenoid and bullous eruptions, and alopecia. Fig. 247 typifies the itchy, scaly, delayed dermatitis associated with long-term gold therapy. It may also resemble lichen planus or pityriasis rosea. Acute allergic reactions, including erythema and urticaria, may also occur.

Fig. 244 Aspirin rash. Urticaria. Rapidly subsided on withdrawing drug.

Fig. 245 Steroid skin changes. Dermal atrophy and pigmentation. Scars due to skin tearing. Permanent.

Fig. 246 Penicillamine rash. Papular erythema. Slowly disappeared on withdrawing drug.

Fig. 247 Gold rash. Scaly, itchy, erythematous patch. Very slowly cleared on withdrawing drug.

**Other drug
side effects**

Some other drug side effects are illustrated here (Figs 248 & 249). Apart from the suspicion that certain drugs are associated with aggravating or even causing peptic ulceration, antirheumatic agents may be associated with other G-I effects, e.g. drug-induced dyspepsia by most of them, constipation due to codeine, diarrhoea due to mefenamic acid, aggravation of colitis by indomethacin, precipitation of pancreatitis by corticosteroids, and induction of malabsorption by colchicine. The widespread iatrogenic influence of antirheumatic drugs on other systems is too extensive to be included here, but should always be borne in mind.

**Problems
related to
nursing and
remedial
therapy**

Iatrogenic disorders may be encountered during nursing or remedial therapy. For example, allergy to local agents or dressings (Fig. 250). Other examples of local disease include burns from lamps used in physiotherapy. More serious iatrogenic effects may arise from improper administration of oral or parenteral drugs.

**Surgical
complications**

One of the most feared complications of rheumatological surgery is immediate or delayed infection. Fig. 251 shows an infected prosthesis which presented many months after surgery. (This may occur despite the most meticulous technique, including the use of local and systemic antibiotics, and specially designed—laminar flow—operating theatres.)

Fig. 248 Perforated peptic ulcer. Patient taking steroids and indomethacin. Note gas under right diaphragm.

Fig. 249 Monilial oesophagitis. Patient taking large doses of antibiotics for septic arthritis.

Fig. 250 Zinc oxide plaster allergy. Patient on leg traction for disc prolapse.

Fig. 251 Infected prosthesis. Note lucent zone around prosthesis/cement outline.